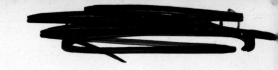

D0967802

AN INTRODUCTION TO

ELECTROCARDIOGRAPHY

AN INTRODUCTION TO
ELECTROCARDIOGRAPHY

L. SCHAMROTH

M.D. (Rand), D.Sc., F.R.C.P. (Edin.),
F.R.C.P. (Glasg.), F.A.C.C., F.R.S. (S.Af.)

Professor of Medicine, University of the Witwatersrand, and
Chief Physician, Baragwanath Hospital, Johannesburg
Republic of South Africa

FIFTH EDITION

BLACKWELL SCIENTIFIC PUBLICATIONS
OXFORD LONDON EDINBURGH MELBOURNE

FIFTH EDITION
© 1976 BLACKWELL SCIENTIFIC PUBLICATIONS

Osney Mead, Oxford OX2 0EL
8 St John Street, London WC1N 2ES
9 Forrest Road, Edinburgh EH1 2QH
P.O. Box 9, North Balwyn, Victoria 3104, Australia

All rights reserved. No part of this publication may be reproduced, stored in a retrieval system, or transmitted, in any form or by any means, electronic, mechanical, photocopying, recording or otherwise without the prior permission of the copyright owner.

ISBN 0 632 08440 5

FIRST PUBLISHED 1957
REPRINTED 1959, 1961
SECOND EDITION 1964
THIRD EDITION 1966
REPRINTED 1968, 1969, 1970
FOURTH EDITION 1973
REPRINTED 1973, 1974
FIFTH EDITION 1976

Japanese translation 1966
Spanish translation 1974
Greek translation 1974

British Library Cataloguing in Publication Data
Schamroth, Leo
  An introduction to electrocardiography.
  5th ed.
  Bibl. –Index.
  ISBN 0–632–08440–5
  1. Title
  616.1'2'0754   RC683.5.E5
  Electrocardiography

Distributed in the United States of America by
J. B. Lippincott Company, Philadelphia
and in Canada by
J. B. Lippincott Company of Canada Ltd. Toronto

Printed in Great Britain at the Alden Press, Oxford

To the Memory of Becky

Contents

PART I. BASIC PRINCIPLES

THE P-QRS-T DEFLECTIONS

PART II. DISORDERS OF CARDIAC RHYTHM

SECTION 1.
BASIC PRINCIPLES

SECTION 2.
DISORDERS OF IMPULSE FORMATION

SECTION 3.

DISORDERS OF IMPULSE CONDUCTION

SECTION 4.

DUAL RHYTHMS

PART III. GENERAL CONSIDERATIONS

The approach to electrocardiographic interpretation. Common associations. Common electrocardiographic manifestations of congenital heart disease. An approach to the diagnosis of arrhythmias. Form for routine reporting.

Foreword

Dr Schamroth publishes this little book on modern electrocardiography at the insistent demand of students and graduates whom he has instructed, and who consider that he should make available for general circulation a method of teaching electrocardiography applicable to clinical practice which is simple, revealing and based upon sound electro-physiological principles.

Simply written, and amply illustrated with many meaningful diagrams, Dr Schamroth's book is a contribution to the rational appreciation and interpretation of electrocardiographic abnormalities by students and practitioners whose training in the physiological aspects of cardiac action has been no more profound than is provided by the undergraduate curriculum.

Present-day literature on electrocardiography is forbidding in its complexity for anyone who has not had specialized training. This book is a welcome addition to electrocardiographic literature, because by its simplicity and correctness it invites understanding.

G. A. ELLIOTT

Professor of Medicine
University of the Witwatersrand
South Africa

Preface to the Fifth Edition

The basic design of this book remains essentially the same as that of the previous editions. It is directed primarily at the beginner, and its aim is simplicity. The emphasis remains on deductive rather than empirical electrocardiographic interpretation.

The whole text has been appreciably revised. New sections have been added on: the hyperacute phase of myocardial infarction, the variant form of angina pectoris (Prinzmetal's Angina), and the hemiblock concept. Many of the diagrams and illustrative electrocardiograms have been replaced, and new ones added.

L. SCHAMROTH

Johannesburg
January 1976

Preface to the First Edition

This volume, it should be stated at the outset, makes no pretensions to be a complete or comprehensive treatise on electrocardiography, nor does it seek to supplant the major works on the subject. It is rather a stepping-stone to the fuller and more detailed study of a most important branch of medical science.

The student, introduced for the first time to the intricacies of electrocardiography, is frequently bewildered, sometimes overwhelmed, by complicated methods of presentation. It is the beginner who has been kept continuously in mind in the writing of this book, and the primary object throughout has been to give him a working knowledge of the subject. Consequently, a certain amount of licence has been taken with a view to clarifying the various processes. Theoretical considerations have been reduced to a minimum, emphasis being placed on the practical aspects. The text has been illustrated as profusely as possible with sketches, a clear drawing invariably being worth pages of script.

Clarity of presentation has thus been the author's aim; if he should succeed in dispersing a few clouds from his readers' minds, his efforts will not have been in vain.

L. SCHAMROTH

Johannesburg
May 1956

Acknowledgements

It is my pleasure to express my thanks to:

Dr William P. Nelson for permission to reproduce his tracing as Fig. 151 in this text.

Dr A. Dubb for permission to reproduce his tracing as Fig. 86 in this text.

The Photographic Department, Department of Medicine, University of the Witwatersrand, for the photographic reproductions.

NOMENCLATURE AND LOCATION OF THE ELECTRODE LEADS

Each electrocardiographic lead has a positive pole or electrode and a negative pole or electrode, which could theoretically be orientated in any relationship to the heart. By convention, however, there are 12 lead placements. These are:

Standard lead I.
Standard lead II.
Standard lead III.
Lead AVR.
Lead AVL.
Lead AVF.
Leads V1 to V6.

Standard leads I, II and III are bipolar leads (see Appendix and Chapter 7).

Leads AVR, AVL, AVF, and V1 to V6 are unipolar leads (see Appendix and Chapter 7).

BASIC ORIENTATION OF THE LEADS

The 12 conventional leads may be divided into two groups, one being orientated in the frontal plane of the body, and the other in the horizontal plane (see Chapter 7 and Fig. 104).

Standard leads I, II and III, and leads AVR, AVL, and AVF are orientated in the **frontal** or **coronal plane** of the body.

The precordial leads—leads V1 to V6—are orientated in the **horizontal plane** of the body.

THE FRONTAL PLANE LEADS

Standard leads I, II, and III
The orientation of the Standard leads is described in Chapter 7.

Unipolar limb leads (see also Chapter 7).
All unipolar leads are termed V leads and consist of extremity or limb leads, and precordial or chest leads. Extremity leads are of low electrical potential and are therefore instrumentally augmented (see Appendix). These augmented extremity leads are prefixed by the letter 'A'.

Lead AVR is the augmented unipolar right arm lead (Fig. 9A). Electrically, the limbs may be viewed as extensions of the torso and it is immaterial whether the electrode is placed on the wrist, arm or shoulder. Thus lead AVR may be considered to 'face' the heart from the right shoulder (Fig. 9B). This lead is usually orientated to the cavity of the heart (see also page 102 and Fig. 105).

Lead AVL is the augmented unipolar left arm lead (Fig. 9A) and may be considered to 'face' the heart from the left shoulder (Fig. 9B). This lead is usually orientated to the anterolateral or superior surface of the left ventricle.

Lead AVF is the augmented unipolar left leg lead (Fig. 9A) and may be considered to 'face' the heart from the left hip (Fig. 9B).

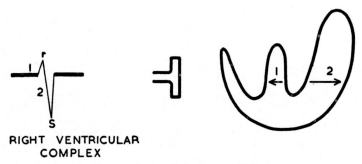

RIGHT VENTRICULAR
COMPLEX

FIG. 10. Precordial, chest or V leads.

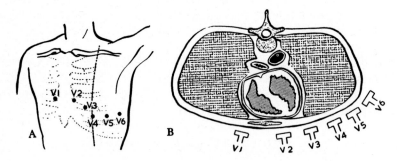

FIG. 11. A transverse representation of the V leads in Fig. 10.

THE HORIZONTAL PLANE LEADS

PRECORDIAL OR CHEST LEADS

The precordial leads are designated by the letter 'V' only (Figs. 10, 11 and 12).

Lead V1 is located over the fourth intercostal space to the right of the sternal border.

Lead V2 is located over the fourth intercostal space to the left of the sternal border.

Lead V3 is located midway between leads V2 and V4.

PART I

Basic Principles

THE P-QRS-T DEFLECTIONS

CHAPTER I

Basic Principles

THE ACTION OF THE GALVANOMETER

When an electrical impulse flows **towards** a unipolar electrode, or the positive electrode of a bipolar lead, the galvanometer will record a **positive** or upward deflection (Diagram A of Fig. 1).

When an electrical impulse flows **away** from a unipolar electrode, or **away** from the positive electrode of a bipolar lead, the galvanometer will record a **negative** or downward deflection (Diagram B of Fig. 1).

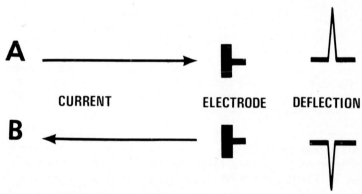

Fig. 1. Diagrams illustrating the effect of current direction on the electrodes of a galvanometer.

THE 'TWO CHAMBER' CONCEPT

It is stating the obvious to say that the heart is a four-chambered organ. It is not often appreciated, however, that, in an electrophysiological sense, the heart consists of only two chambers: one formed by the atria, and the other formed by the ventricles (Fig. 2). The two atria function as a single physiological chamber—an electrophysiological unit: there is no electrical boundary between them, and both are activated by a single activation process. This functional electrophysiological unit may be referred to as the **bi-atrial chamber.** Similarly, the ventricles also function as an electrophysiological unit, which may be referred to as the

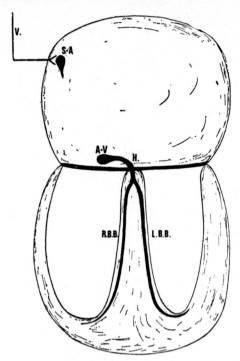

FIG. 2. Diagrammatic representation of the two electrophysiological chambers. V. = vagus nerve. S-A = sino-atrial node. A-V = atrio-ventricular node. H = bundle of His. R.B.B. = right bundle branch. L.B.B. = left bundle branch.

biventricular chamber. The two electrophysiological chambers are separated from each other by an electrically inert conduction barrier formed by the fibrous A-V ring. Communication across this barrier under normal circumstances is only possible through the specialized conducting system formed by the A-V node, the bundle of His, the bundle branches and their ramifications.

THE DOMINANCE OF THE LEFT VENTRICLE

The free wall of the left ventricle, and the interventricular septum have relatively thick walls (large muscle masses) and together constitute a uniform ring of muscle or chamber—the anatomical left ventricle (Fig. 3). It is quite evident from a cross-section of the ventricles that the interventricular septum and the free wall of the left ventricle constitute an anatomical continuum (Fig. 3). The free wall of the right ventricle is, in effect, merely a thin anatomical appendage of the left ventricle.

The interventricular septum also contracts functionally with the free

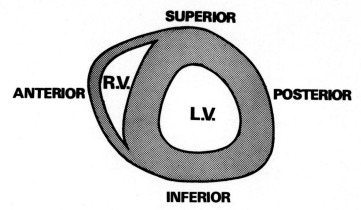

F𝐼G. 3. Diagrammatic representation of a cross-section through the ventricles.

wall of the left ventricle, constituting the main haemodynamic pump of the heart. The right ventricle functions principally as a conduit.

From the electrocardiological viewpoint, the left ventricle is also the dominant chamber. For example, anterior wall myocardial infarction refers principally to infarction of the interventricular septum. The interventricular septum thus, in effect, constitutes the 'electrical' anterior wall of the biventricular chamber, whereas the thin free wall of the right ventricle constitutes the anatomical anterior wall of the biventricular chamber.

THE MODES OF ATRIAL AND VENTRICULAR ACTIVATION

The bi-atrial chamber is a relatively thin-walled structure and is not equipped with the highly specialized conducting system of the ventricles. Activation of the bi-atrial chamber therefore occurs **longitudinally** and by **contiguity**, spreading from its point of origin in the S-A node to engulf the whole chamber, each fibre in turn activating the adjacent fibre (Diagram A of Fig. 4).

Activation of the ventricles is effected through the specialized and highly efficient conducting system which transmits the supraventricular impulse very rapidly to all the endocardial regions of the chamber. The muscle is then activated from endocardial to epicardial surfaces through the terminal ramifications of the conducting system. Excitation therefore occurs **transversely** through the ventricular myocardium, and this enables the whole chamber to be activated near-synchronously (Diagram B of Fig. 4).

These different forms of activation have both physiological and inter-

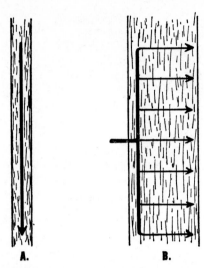

FIG. 4. Diagrams illustrating: (A) the mode of atrial activation. (B) the mode of ventricular activation.

pretative connotations. For example, atrial hypertrophy cannot be diagnosed electrocardiographically since the longitudinal form of atrial activation can only reflect *atrial enlargement*. The transverse form of ventricular activation, however, does permit electrocardiographic connotation with ventricular hypertrophy.

THE NOMENCLATURE OF THE ELECTROCARDIOGRAPHIC DEFLECTIONS

The electrocardiographic deflections are arbitrarily and sequentially named P, QRS, T and U. The P wave reflects atrial activation. The QRS complex reflects ventricular activation. The T wave reflects ventricular recovery. The genesis of the U wave is still controversial.

Note: An initial downward deflection after the P wave is termed a *q* wave. An initial upward deflection after the P wave is termed an *r* wave. The ensuing deflections are named by the succeeding alphabetical letters.

ACTIVATION OF THE VENTRICLES

In an electrocardiological sense, the ventricles are composed of three muscle masses: the interventricular septum, the free wall of the right ventricle (the right ventricular muscle mass), the free wall of the left ventricle (the left ventricular muscle mass) (Fig. 5).

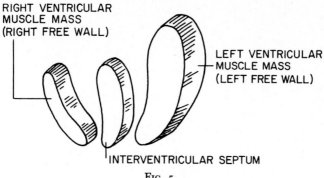

RIGHT VENTRICULAR
MUSCLE MASS
(RIGHT FREE WALL)

LEFT VENTRICULAR
MUSCLE MASS
(LEFT FREE WALL)

INTERVENTRICULAR SEPTUM

FIG. 5.

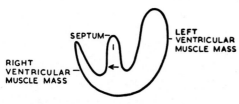

SEPTUM

LEFT
VENTRICULAR
MUSCLE MASS

RIGHT
VENTRICULAR
MUSCLE MASS

FIG. 6. First stage of depolarization.

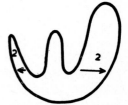

FIG. 7. Second stage of
depolarization.

Activation or depolarization of the ventricles begins in the left side of the interventricular septum and spreads through the septum from left to right (arrow 1 in Fig. 6).

Depolarization then proceeds outwards *simultaneously* through the free walls of both ventricles from endocardial to epicardial surfaces (arrows labelled 2 in Fig. 7).

The free wall of the left ventricle has a larger muscle mass—and hence a larger potential electrical force—than the free wall of the right ventricle (Figs. 3 and 5). Consequently, as depolarization of both free walls occurs simultaneously, the larger left ventricular forces counteract the smaller right ventricular forces. The result is a single force directed from right to left (arrow 2 in Fig. 8). Thus, *for convenience*, depolarization of the ventricles may be represented in simplified form as a small initial force from left to right through the septum, followed by a larger force from right to left through the free wall of the left ventricle (Fig. 8).

An electrode orientated to the left ventricle (e.g. lead V6 in Fig. 8) will record a small initial downward deflection (a small q wave) caused by the spread of the stimulus *away* from the electrode through the septum, followed by a larger upward deflection (a tall R wave) caused by the spread of the stimulus *towards* the electrode through the left

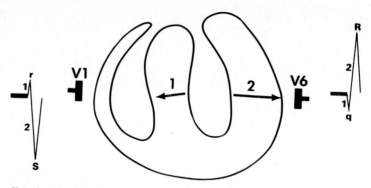

FIG. 8. Diagrammatic representation of the basic form of ventricular depolarization and its effect on leads V1 and V6.

ventricular muscle mass (Fig. 8). The result is a qR complex (e.g. leads AVL, V5 and V6 in Fig. 71).

Conversely, an electrode orientated to the right ventricle (e.g. lead V1 in Fig. 8), will record a small initial upright deflection (a small r wave) caused by the spread of the stimulus *towards* the electrode through the septum, followed by a larger downward deflection (a deep S wave) caused by the spread of the stimulus *away* from the electrode through the left ventricular muscle mass (Fig. 8). The result is an rS complex (e.g. leads V1 and V2 in Fig. 71).

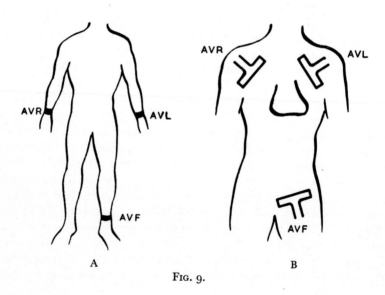

FIG. 9.

NOMENCLATURE AND LOCATION OF THE ELECTRODE LEADS

Each electrocardiographic lead has a positive pole or electrode and a negative pole or electrode, which could theoretically be orientated in any relationship to the heart. By convention, however, there are 12 lead placements. These are:

Standard lead I.
Standard lead II.
Standard lead III.
Lead AVR.
Lead AVL.
Lead AVF.
Leads V1 to V6.

Standard leads I, II and III are bipolar leads (see Appendix and Chapter 7).

Leads AVR, AVL, AVF, and V1 to V6 are unipolar leads (see Appendix and Chapter 7).

BASIC ORIENTATION OF THE LEADS

The 12 conventional leads may be divided into two groups, one being orientated in the frontal plane of the body, and the other in the horizontal plane (see Chapter 7 and Fig. 104).

Standard leads I, II and III, and leads AVR, AVL, and AVF are orientated in the **frontal** or **coronal plane** of the body.

The precordial leads—leads V1 to V6—are orientated in the **horizontal plane** of the body.

THE FRONTAL PLANE LEADS

Standard leads I, II, and III
The orientation of the Standard leads is described in Chapter 7.

Unipolar limb leads (see also Chapter 7).
All unipolar leads are termed V leads and consist of extremity or limb leads, and precordial or chest leads. Extremity leads are of low electrical potential and are therefore instrumentally augmented (see Appendix). These augmented extremity leads are prefixed by the letter 'A'.

Lead AVR is the augmented unipolar right arm lead (Fig. 9A). Electrically, the limbs may be viewed as extensions of the torso and it is immaterial whether the electrode is placed on the wrist, arm or shoulder. Thus lead AVR may be considered to 'face' the heart from the right shoulder (Fig. 9B). This lead is usually orientated to the cavity of the heart (see also page 102 and Fig. 105).

Lead AVL is the augmented unipolar left arm lead (Fig. 9A) and may be considered to 'face' the heart from the left shoulder (Fig. 9B). This lead is usually orientated to the anterolateral or superior surface of the left ventricle.

Lead AVF is the augmented unipolar left leg lead (Fig. 9A) and may be considered to 'face' the heart from the left hip (Fig. 9B).

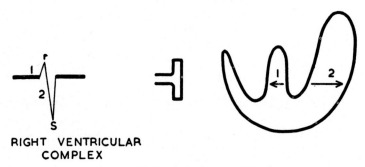

RIGHT   VENTRICULAR
COMPLEX

FIG. 10. Precordial, chest or V leads.

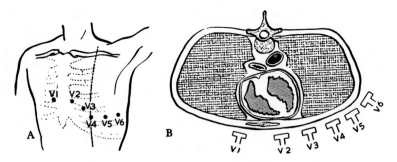

FIG. 11. A transverse representation of the V leads in Fig. 10.

THE HORIZONTAL PLANE LEADS

PRECORDIAL OR CHEST LEADS

The precordial leads are designated by the letter 'V' only (Figs. 10, 11 and 12).

Lead V1 is located over the fourth intercostal space to the right of the sternal border.

Lead V2 is located over the fourth intercostal space to the left of the sternal border.

Lead V3 is located midway between leads V2 and V4.

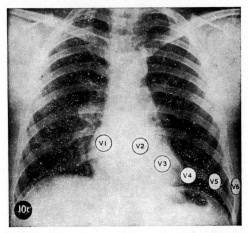

FIG. 12. The V leads and their relationship to the heart and thorax.

Lead V4 is located on the midclavicular line over the fifth interspace.

Lead V5 is located on the anterior axillary line at the same level as lead V4.

Lead V6 is located over the midaxillary line at the same level as leads V4 and V5.

ORIENTATION OF THE ELECTROCARDIOGRAPHIC LEADS TO THE LEFT VENTRICULAR 'CONE'

Since the left ventricle is the dominant chamber of the heart, orientation of the electrodes to this chamber is of particular importance. The left ventricle is in the form of a cone whose apex is directed downward

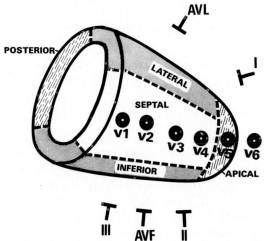

FIG. 13. Diagrammatic representation of the various surfaces of the left ventricular anatomical cone, and their relationship to the frontal and horizontal plane leads.

and to the left (Fig. 13). It has five surfaces or regions each with a specific lead orientation. Thus:

Surface or region	Lead orientation
1. Anteroseptal	Leads V1 to V4.
2. Anterolateral or superior	Standard lead I and lead AVL.
3. Inferior	Standard leads II and III, and lead AVF.
4. Posterior	No direct lead orientation. Diagnosis of abnormality in this region is made from inverse or 'mirror-image' changes in leads V1 to V4.
5. Apical	Leads V5 and V6.

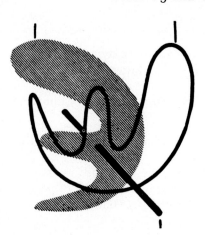

FIG. 14. Rotation round the anteroposterior axis.

THE ELECTROCARDIOGRAPHIC REFLECTION OF THE ANATOMICAL HEART POSITION

'ROTATION' OF THE HEART

It was previously thought that the anatomical orientation of the heart could vary under both normal and pathological conditions, and that this could be reflected electrocardiographically. It is very doubtful, however, whether true movement does indeed occur. It is far more likely that so-called clockwise and counter-clockwise rotation, and horizontal and vertical heart positions reflect changes in mean frontal and horizontal plane electrical axes—a change in the orientation of the mean electrical force rather than a change in anatomical position. Nevertheless, the terms are still in use, and the concept is presented here for didactic purposes with the aforementioned reservation in mind.

The heart can theoretically 'rotate' around two hypothetical axes: the *anteroposterior axis* and the *oblique or longitudinal axis*. 'Rotation' around the anteroposterior axis reflects rotation in the frontal plane. 'Rotation' around the oblique or longitudinal axis reflects rotation in the horizontal plane.

'ROTATION' IN THE FRONTAL PLANE

The anteroposterior axis runs through the septum of the heart from anterior to posterior surfaces (Fig. 14). Rotation around this axis will result in a horizontal or vertical heart position, and is diagnosed from the presence of a dominantly positive QRS deflection or qR complex in lead AVL or lead AVF.

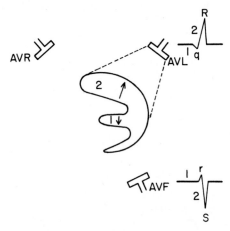

FIG. 15. Horizontal heart position—a qR complex in lead AVL.

'HORIZONTAL' POSITION

In the 'horizontal' position the main muscle mass of the left ventricle is orientated upwards and to the left, i.e. towards lead AVL and the positive pole of Standard lead I (Fig. 15). These leads will therefore record a qR or 'left ventricular' complex (e.g. lead AVL in Fig. 71).

'VERTICAL' POSITION

In the 'vertical' position the main muscle mass of the left ventricle is orientated downwards and to the left, i.e. towards lead AVF and the positive pole of Standard lead II (Fig. 16). These leads will therefore record a qR or 'left ventricular' complex (e.g. lead AVF in Fig. 73).

SUMMARY

A qR complex in lead AVL and Standard lead I indicates a **'horizontal'** heart position.

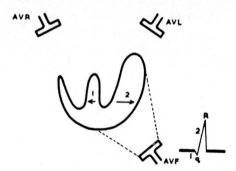

FIG. 16. Vertical position of the heart.

A qR complex in lead AVF and Standard lead II indicates a **'vertical'** heart position.

Comment: It must be stressed once again that it is doubtful whether any marked movement or rotation does, in fact, occur in this plane. Slight anatomical shifts do occur with respiratory excursion, and some 'horizontality' of the heart may result from upward displacement due to ascites or pregnancy. Marked 'horizontality' of the heart, however, most likely reflects left axis deviation; and this is not the expression of heart movement, but rather an intraventricular conduction defect (see Chapter 7).

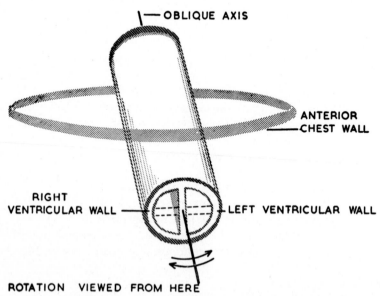

FIG. 17. Diagrammatic representation of the heart with the apex removed, to show rotation round the oblique axis.

'ROTATION' IN THE HORIZONTAL PLANE

The oblique or longitudinal axis of the heart runs obliquely from the apex to the base of the heart (Fig. 17). Rotation round this axis is conventionally viewed from below the heart looking towards the apex and will result in clockwise or counter-clockwise movement. This is diagnosed from the precordial leads.

CLOCKWISE ROTATION

Clockwise rotation round the oblique axis will cause the right ventricle to assume an anterior position. The right ventricle and interventricular septum will lie parallel to and face the anterior chest wall and the V

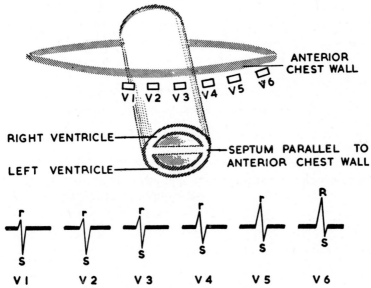

FIG. 18. Extreme clockwise rotation (diagrammatic).

leads (Fig. 18). Leads V1–V6 thus face the right ventricle and record rS or 'right ventricular' complexes (Fig. 77).

COUNTER-CLOCKWISE ROTATION

Counter-clockwise rotation about the oblique axis of the heart causes the left ventricle to rotate a few degrees anteriorly so that both right and left ventricles face the anterior chest wall and the precordial leads (Fig. 19). As a result, leads V1–V3 face the right ventricle and record Sr complexes; leads V4–V6 face the left ventricle and record qR complexes (Fig. 70). The area of change from rS to qR pattern is known as the **transition zone**.

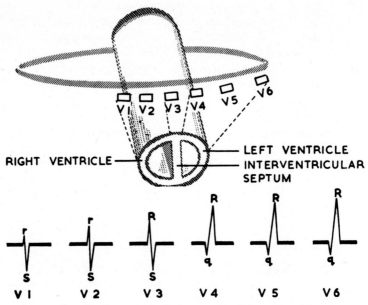

FIG. 19. Counter-clockwise rotation (diagrammatic).

SUMMARY

Clockwise rotation: rS complexes in leads V1 to V6.

Counter-clockwise rotation: rS complexes in leads V1, V2, (V3), qR complexes in leads (V3), V4, V5, V6.

CHAPTER 2

Myocardial Death, Injury and Ischaemia

MYOCARDIAL INFARCTION

Myocardial infarction is reflected electrocardiographically by the electrocardiographic parameters of *necrosis, injury* and *ischaemia*. The infarction process progresses through three phases:

1. **An early 'hyperacute' phase.**
2. **A fully evolved phase.**
3. **A phase of resolution.**

The principles governing the electrocardiographic manifestations of necrosis, injury and ischaemia are best illustrated with reference to the fully evolved phase, and this will be considered first.

THE FULLY EVOLVED PHASE OF ACUTE MYOCARDIAL INFARCTION

THE ELECTROCARDIOGRAPHIC MANIFESTATION OF MYOCARDIAL NECROSIS

Myocardial necrosis is reflected by a **deep and wide Q wave** in electrodes orientated towards the necrotic area.

Mechanism
Dead tissue is electrically inert and cannot be activated or depolarized. If the dead tissue involves the full thickness of the muscle wall it constitutes a transmural infarct (Diagram A of Fig. 20) and there is, in an electrical sense, a 'hole' or 'window' in the muscle wall (Diagram B of Fig. 20).

An electrode orientated to or placed over this 'hole' reflects activity of distant healthy muscle as 'seen' through the 'window' (Fig. 21).

Thus an electrode placed over an area of dead muscle in the left ventricular wall reflects firstly septal depolarization—a negative deflection (arrow 1 in Fig. 21) and, secondly, distant right ventricular depolarization—a further negative deflection (arrow 2 in Fig. 21).

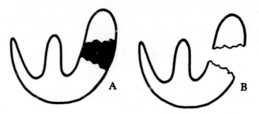

FIG. 20. (A) Diagrammatic illustration of the dead tissue of a transmural infarct. (B) The 'electrical hole' or 'window' created by the dead tissue.

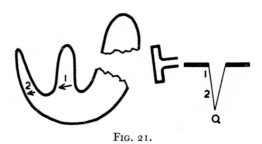

FIG. 21.

This results in a broad deep Q wave—the pathological Q wave of myocardial infarction (e.g. leads V2, V3 and V4 of Fig. 28).

Note: An entirely negative deflection without an ensuing R wave is sometimes termed a QS deflection.

This phenomenon may also be interpreted vectorially, in the sense that **electrical forces tend to move away from a necrotic or infarcted area** (see also Chapter 7, page 106).

THE ELECTROCARDIOGRAPHIC MANIFESTATION OF MYOCARDIAL INJURY

Myocardial injury is reflected electrocardiographically by **deviation of the S-T segment**. The S-T segment is, so to speak, *deviated towards the surface of the injured tissue*. Thus, if the injury is dominantly epicardial (as illustrated in Diagram A of Fig. 22), the S-T segment is deviated towards the injured epicardial surface, and a lead orientated towards this surface (e.g. lead V6 in Diagram A of Fig. 22) will reflect a raised S-T segment. Conversely, a lead orientated towards the uninjured surface (e.g. lead AVR in Diagram A of Fig. 22) will reflect a depressed S-T segment. With a dominantly subendocardial injury, a lead orientated to the injured subendocardial surface (e.g. lead AVR in Diagram B of

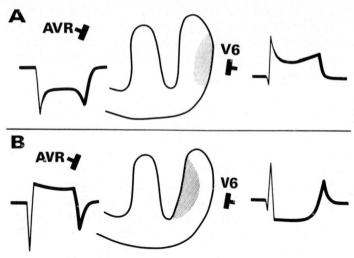

FIG. 22. Diagrams illustrating the deviation of the S-T segment in: (A) dominant subepicardial injury, and (B) dominant subendocardial injury.

Fig. 22) will reflect an elevated S-T segment, whereas a lead orientated to the uninjured surface (lead V6 in Diagram B of Fig. 22) will reflect a depressed S-T segment.

Since the myocardial injury in most infarctions is dominantly epicardial with some subendocardial 'sparing' (Fig. 23), the manifestation presents electrocardiographically with elevated S-T segments in leads

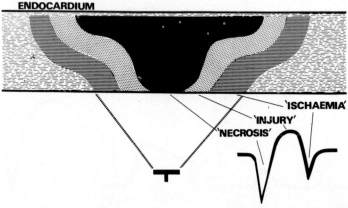

FIG. 23. An idealized representation of the combined patterns of the fully evolved phase of acute myocardial infarction. The infarct is pyramid-shaped with a broad base towards the endocardium. The diagram also illustrates the hypothetical 'rind' of subendocardial 'sparing' (see Appendix, page 229).

orientated to the epicardial surface. The S-T segments in the fully evolved phase of the infarction are, in addition, *coved or convex-upward*.

The mechanism of these S-T segment shifts is still controversial. Several theories have been propounded, one of which is considered in the Appendix (page 228).

THE ELECTROCARDIOGRAPHIC EFFECTS OF MYOCARDIAL ISCHAEMIA

Myocardial ischaemia is reflected by an inverted T wave in leads orientated to the ischaemic surface. Inverted T waves are, however, non-specific and may be associated with many other conditions both normal and abnormal. However, the T waves associated with myocardial ischaemia have certain characteristics which tend to reflect their 'ischaemic' origin. They are usually **'arrowhead'** in appearance being *peaked* and *symmetrical* (e.g. leads V2 to V6 in Fig. 28).

THE COMBINED PATTERNS OF THE FULLY EVOLVED PHASE OF MYOCARDIAL INFARCTION

A severely infarcted area consists of necrotic tissue surrounded by a zone of injured tissue which, in turn, is surrounded by a zone of ischaemic tissue (Fig. 23).

A conventional electrode cannot be pinpointed or placed directly over the heart muscle itself; it is situated some distance away and therefore subtends a relatively large area to include the zones of necrotic, injured and ischaemic tissues (Fig. 23). Such an electrode will record all three patterns, viz. the pathological Q wave, the raised coved S-T segment and the inverted, pointed symmetrical T wave (Diagram C of Fig. 24 and leads V2 to V4 in Fig. 28). This will be referred to as the *typical infarction pattern*.

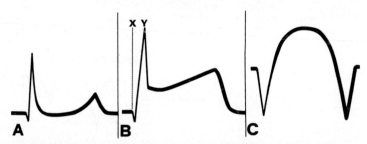

Fig. 24. Diagrams illustrating: (A) normal QRST complex, (B) the hyperacute phase of myocardial infarction, and (C) the fully evolved phase of myocardial infarction. Interval X–Y represents the increased ventricular activation time.

An electrode orientated towards injured and ischaemic tissue but not necrotic tissue will record the raised, coved S-T segment and the inverted pointed symmetrical T wave only. The pathological q wave might be absent or relatively insignificant (e.g. lead V6 of Fig. 28).

Note: Reciprocal depression of the S-T segment will occur in leads orientated towards the uninjured surface. However, the diagnosis of infarction must not be based on depressed S-T segments only, as these may occur in conditions such as angina pectoris (see page 39). *The diagnosis must be based on pathological Q waves and/or the typically raised and coved S-T segments.*

THE HYPERACUTE PHASE OF MYOCARDIAL INFARCTION

The hyperacute phase of myocardial infarction occurs within the few hours of the onset of myocardial infarction. It was so named to distinguish it from the well-recognized fully evolved phase of myocardial infarction, as described earlier in this chapter. The condition has received insufficient emphasis in the electrocardiographic literature. Furthermore, since the transition to the fully evolved phase occurs relatively early—usually within 24 hours, the manifestation is not infrequently missed. Thus, the first electrocardiogram of the patient is often recorded during the fully evolved phase. Yet, the hyperacute phase is probably the most important and critical developmental stage of the infarction process, for it is then that the complication of primary ventricular fibrillation is most likely to occur. In other words, the manifestation of the hyperacute phase is an indication for intense vigilance and the necessity for coronary care monitoring.

ELECTROCARDIOGRAPHIC MANIFESTATIONS
The hyperacute phase of myocardial infarction is characterized by the following three principal electrocardiographic manifestations in leads orientated to the infarcted surface (Diagram B of Fig. 24, and Figs. 25 and 26):

1. *Slope-elevation of the S-T segment*
The S-T segment is elevated—often markedly so—and has a straight upward slope to the apex of the T wave. The slope may also be slightly concave-upward. The S-T segment thus blends smoothly and imperceptibly with the proximal limb of the tall and widened T wave (see below).

Leads orientated to the uninjured surface usually reflect marked reciprocal S-T segment depression.

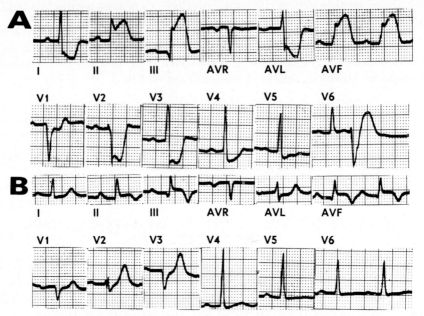

FIG. 25. Electrocardiogram A was recorded on admission to the coronary care unit, and shows the hyperacute early injury phase of acute inferior wall myocardial infarction. This is reflected by the following:

(a) There is marked slope-elevation of the S-T segments in Standard leads II and III, and lead AVF.

(b) There is an increase in the amplitude of the R wave in Standard leads II and III, and lead AVF (compare with Electrocardiogram B).

(c) There is an increase in ventricular activation time, as reflected by a delay in the inscription of the intrinsicoid deflection to 0.06 sec in Standard lead III and lead AVF.

(d) There is a reciprocal depression of the S-T segment in leads V1 to V5, Standard lead I and lead AVL.

(e) The single ventricular extrasystole in lead V6 reflects a primary S-T segment change. This is reflected by the upward coving of the S-T segment instead of the straight or minimally concave-upward secondary S-T segment change of uncomplicated ventricular extrasystole.

(f) The low to inverted T waves in leads V5 and V6 reflect a lateral extension of the myocardial ischaemia.

(g) There is first-degree A-V block, the P-R interval measures 0.24 sec.

Electrocardiogram B was recorded 2 days later when the patient no longer had any chest pain and shows the fully evolved phase of acute inferior wall myocardial infarction. This is reflected by the following:

(a) The S-T segments are coved and elevated, and the T waves are inverted, sharply pointed and arrowhead in appearance in Standard leads II and III, and leaf AVF.

(b) Standard lead III has a pathological Q wave.

(c) The T waves are low to inverted in leads V5 and V6, representing some lateral, apical, extension of the myocardial ischaemia.

(d) Standard lead I, lead AVL and leads V1 to V3 reflect reciprocal, symmetrical and widened T waves.

(e) There is first degree A-V block, the P-R interval measures 0.24 sec.

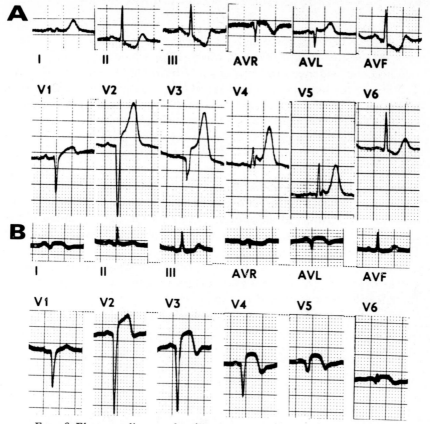

FIG. 26. Electrocardiogram showing acute extensive anterior wall myocardial infarction and left posterior hemiblock.

Electrocardiogram A shows the very early hyperacute phase of acute
anterior wall myocardial infarction. This is reflected by the very tall
T waves in leads V2 to V6, Standard lead I and lead AVL. There is
also a degree of slope-elevation of the S-T segments in leads V2 to V4
and lead AVL.

Standard leads II and III and lead AVF reflect reciprocal depression
of the S-T segments. This is the mirror-image pattern of the S-T segment slope-elevation and the inverted T waves.

The QS complexes of myocardial necrosis are present in leads V2 and
V3, reflecting a loss of the initial positivity. Note that the initial small r
wave is still present in lead V1, but has disappeared in leads V2 and V3.

Note: Very tall and wide T waves are, at times, the earliest and most
striking manifestations of acute myocardial infarction.

Electrocardiogram B shows the fully evolved phase of the acute
extensive anterior wall myocardial infarction. The parameters of myocardial necrosis are reflected by the QS complexes in leads V1 to V5,
Standard lead I and lead AVL, and the pathological Q wave of the Qr
complex in lead V6. The parameters of myocardial injury and
ischaemia are reflected by the coved and elevated S-T segments and
inverted, symmetrical T waves in leads V2 to V6, Standard lead I and
lead AVL.

The left posterior hemiblock is reflected by the mean frontal plane
QRS axis of +90° to +100°.

2. *Tall and widened T wave*

The T wave becomes appreciably taller and may approach, or at times even exceed, the height of the R wave (Figs. 25 and 26). The T wave also becomes widened, and its proximal limb blends with the elevated S-T segment (see above), so that the two components cannot be separated. These very tall T waves may, at times, be the dominant feature of the hyperacute phase of myocardial infarction.

The classic pathological Q wave of myocardial infarction does not occur until this large amplitude T wave has regressed.

3. *Increased ventricular activation time*

There is an increase in the ventricular activation time, i.e. a delay in the onset of the intrinsicoid deflection: the time from the beginning of the QRS complex to the apex of the R wave (interval X–Y in Diagram B of Fig. 24; see also Fig. 199).

This manifestation is due to a degree of intraventricular—injury—block: the activation process takes longer to travel through the injured though still viable infarcted region.

The QRS complex may occasionally be increased in amplitude.

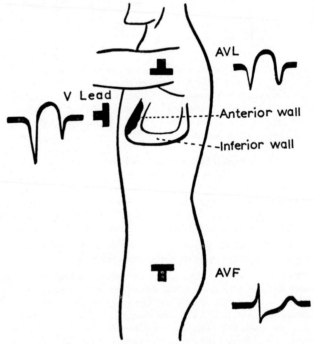

FIG. 27. Anterior myocardial infarction.

Note: The hyperacute phase of myocardial infarction is analogous to the manifestation of the variant form of angina pectoris where it occurs as a transient phenomenon (see page 41).

LOCALIZATION OF INFARCTED AREAS

Infarcts occur predominantly in the anterior, inferior (or diaphragmatic), and posterior, walls of the left ventricle (Figs. 27, 29, 30, 31, 33, 35, 37 and 38; see also Fig. 13).

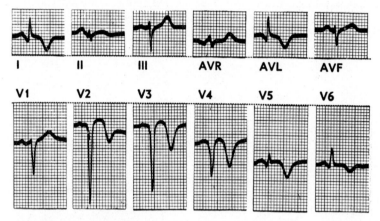

FIG. 28. Electrocardiogram showing the fully evolved phase of acute extensive anterior myocardial infarction. Note the typical infarction pattern in leads V2 to V6, AVL and Standard lead I.

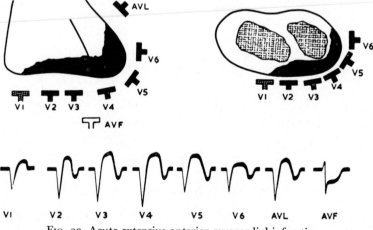

FIG. 29. Acute extensive anterior myocardial infarction.

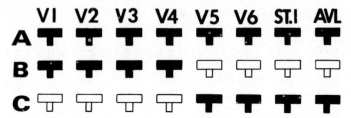

FIG. 30. Diagrams illustrating the classification of anterior infarction. Leads with the blackened electrodes reflect the infarction pattern. (A) Extensive anterior infarction. (B) Anteroseptal infarction. (C) Anterolateral infarction.

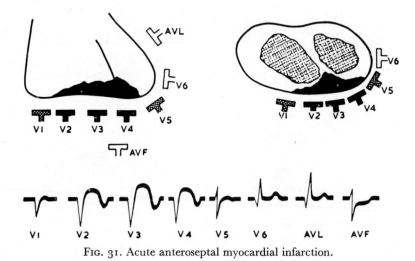

FIG. 31. Acute anteroseptal myocardial infarction.

ANTERIOR WALL INFARCTION

The anterior surface of the left ventricle is orientated towards the precordial leads (Figs. 27 and 37); the anterolateral surface of the left

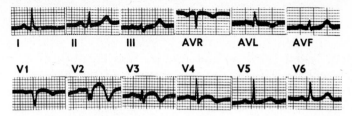

FIG. 32. Electrocardiogram showing the fully evolved phase of anteroseptal infarction. This is reflected by the pathological Q waves in leads
V1 to V3, the coved elevated S-T segments and the inverted T waves in
leads V1 to V4.

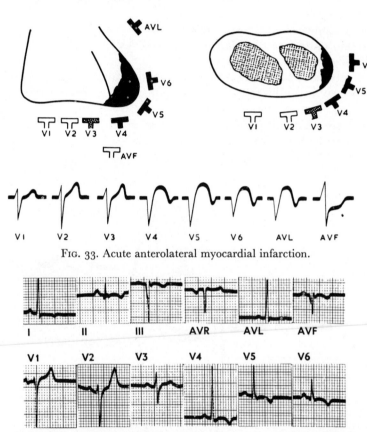

FIG. 33. Acute anterolateral myocardial infarction.

FIG. 34. Electrocardiogram showing regressing inferolateral wall myocardial infarction. The electrocardiogram was recorded 3 weeks after
the onset of acute myocardial infarction. The necrosis of the inferior
wall is reflected by the pathological Q waves in Standard lead II and
lead AVF as well as the prominent q wave in Standard lead II. The
myocardial injury and ischaemia are reflected by the slightly elevated
and coved S-T segments, and the inverted T waves in Standard leads
II and III, and lead AVF. The anterolateral extension is reflected by
the coved S-T segments and inverted T waves in leads V4 to V6 and
Standard lead I, as well as the inverted T wave in lead AVL.

ventricle is orientated towards lead AVL and the positive pole of Standard lead I (Figs. 29 and 106; see also Fig. 13). Thus anterior infarcts will be reflected by the presence of the typical infarction pattern—pathological Q wave, raised S-T segment and inverted T wave—in Standard lead I, lead AVL and the precordial leads (Figs. 27, 28, 29 and 30).

Anterior infarcts may be further arbitrarily divided into **extensive anterior infarction** (Figs. 28, 29 and 30); **anteroseptal infarction** (Figs. 30, 31 and 32); and **anterolateral infarction** (Figs. 30, 33 and 34).

An **extensive anterior infarction** is reflected by the typical infarction pattern in Standard lead I, lead AVL and *all* the precordial leads (Figs. 26, 28, 29 and 30).

An **anteroseptal infarction** is an infarction across the interventricular septum and is reflected by the typical infarction pattern in leads V1 to V4 (Figs. 30, 31 and 32).

An **anterolateral infarction** is reflected by the typical infarction pattern in leads I, AVL, and in leads V4 to V6 (Figs. 30, 33 and 34).

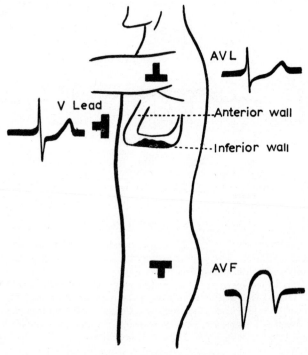

FIG. 35. Inferior myocardial infarction.

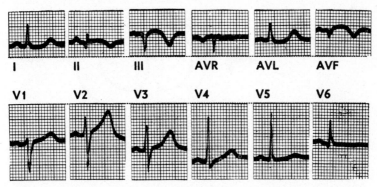

FIG. 36. Electrocardiogram showing the fully evolved phase of acute inferior myocardial infarction. Note the typical infarction pattern in Standard leads II and III and lead AVF. Leads AVL and Standard I show reciprocal S-T segment depression. The T waves are low in leads V5 and V6 suggesting some anterolateral extension.

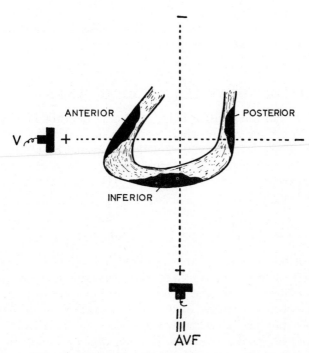

FIG. 37. Diagram illustrating the location of anterior, inferior and posterior myocardial infarctions.

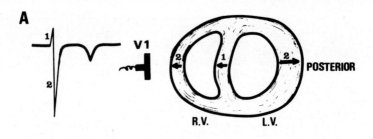

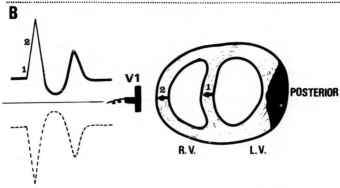

FIG. 38. Diagrams illustrating (A) normal ventricular depolarization, and (B) ventricular depolarization during true posterior infarction (see text).

INFERIOR—DIAPHRAGMATIC—INFARCTION

Lead AVF and the positive poles of Standard Leads II and III are orientated to the inferior or diaphragmatic surface of the heart (Figs. 35 and 37). Thus, inferior infarcts will be reflected by the presence of the typical infarction pattern—pathological Q wave, raised S-T segment and inverted T wave—in leads II, III and AVF (Figs. 25, 34, 36, 39 and 111).

TRUE POSTERIOR INFARCTION

Infarction of the true posterior wall of the left ventricle is uncommon and manifests with distinctive electrocardiographic features which are strikingly different from the usual infarction pattern. The classic electrocardiographic features of the fully evolved phase of acute myocardial infarction, viz. deep and wide Q wave, elevated and coved S-T segment, and inverted arrowhead T wave, which manifest in the conventional leads orientated to the infarcted surface, do not occur. This is because none of these leads is orientated towards the true posterior sur-

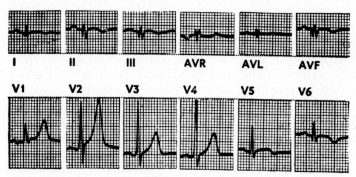

FIG. 39. Electrocardiogram showing the features of inferolateral myo-cardial infarction with true posterior extension. The infarction pattern is seen in Standard leads II and III, and lead AVF, indicating the presence of an inferior infarction. The infarction pattern is also seen in lead V6 indicating lateral extension. The tall R wave and tall sym-metrical T wave in leads V1 and V2 indicates true posterior extension.

face of the heart. The diagnosis of true posterior infarction is thus made from 'inverse' changes in leads which are orientated towards the un-injured—anterior—surface of the heart, viz. leads V1 and V2 (see also Fig. 13).

ELECTROCARDIOGRAPHIC MANIFESTATIONS OF TRUE POSTERIOR INFARCTION

True posterior infarction manifests electrocardiographically with:

1. *Tall and slightly widened R waves in leads V1 and V2.*[4, 29]
2. *Tall, wide and symmetrical T waves in leads V1 and V2.*
3. *Slightly depressed, concave-upward S-T segments in leads V1 and V2.*

The genesis of these changes is considered below.

1. Tall and slightly widened R waves in leads V1 and V2[4, 29]

Depolarization of the normal heart begins in the left side of the inter-ventricular septum and spreads from left to right—and anteriorly—through the septum (Vector 1 in Diagram A of Fig. 38). This is followed by simultaneous activation from endocardial to epicardial surfaces of the free walls of the right (anterior) and left (posterior) ventricles (Vectors 2 in Diagram A of Fig. 38). Since, however, the left or posterior wall has a larger muscle mass, and hence a larger potential electrical force, its activation force will counteract the smaller force of the right (anterior) ventricle which is opposite in direction. This is reflected in leads V1 and V2 by a small initial r wave—caused by the 'septal' force moving toward the electrode, followed by a deep S wave resulting from the left or posterior wall force moving away from the electrode.

When the posterior wall is infarcted, the left or posterior wall force is lost (Diagram B of Fig. 38). Thus, activation of the interventricular septum (Vector 1 in Diagram B of Fig. 38) is followed by activation of the free or anterior wall of the right ventricle. Both forces are now orientated towards leads V1 and V2 resulting in tall and widened R waves in these leads. This may also be expressed as an increase in the R/S ratio to greater than 1 (normal being less than 1). This manifestation is, in effect, a mirror-image of the pathologic Q wave which would be recorded by an electrode orientated towards the posterior surface of the heart (dotted lines in Diagram B of Fig. 38).

There are, however, other conditions which give rise to tall R waves in leads V1 and V2 which must be excluded before the diagnosis of true posterior infarction can be established with certainty. These are:

(a) *Right ventricular dominance* (see page 70).
(b) *The Wolff-Parkinson-White syndrome* (see page 195).
(c) *Certain forms of right bundle branch block.*

These may be excluded by the associated electrocardiographic features —for example, the presence of a delta wave in the Wolff-Parkinson-White syndrome, the RsR' pattern of right bundle branch block, and the right axis deviation and associated right atrial enlargement of right ventricular dominance. Moreover, true posterior infarction is usually associated with tall symmetrical T waves in the right precordial leads (see below) whereas the other conditions are not.

2. Tall, upright, and symmetrical T waves in leads V1 and V2

The T wave vector is always directed away from the area of infarction. Thus, in true posterior infarction, the T wave vector is directed anteriorly, resulting in tall, symmetrical T waves in leads V1 and V2.

3. Depression of the S-T segment in leads V1 and V2

In acute myocardial infarction, the S-T segment vector shifts towards the injured surface, i.e. to leads orientated to the injured surface which reflect elevated and coved S-T segments. In the case of true posterior infarction, the S-T segment vector will thus shift away from leads orientated towards the anterior surface of the heart, thereby resulting in depressed and concave-upward S-T segments in leads V1 and V2. Note that the S-T segment depression is not usually marked, and the S-T segment may, in fact, be isoelectric (Fig. 39).

THE 'INVERSE' CHANGES
The combination of tall R waves, depressed S-T segments, and tall,

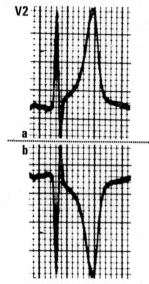

FIG. 40. (a) Enlargement of lead V2 of Fig. 39 showing tall R wave and tall symmetrical T wave. (b) Mirror-image of lead V2 showing deep broad 'Q wave' and deep symmetrical 'T wave'.

symmetrical T waves in the right precordial leads occurring in true posterior myocardial infarction is, in effect, the mirror-image of the typical infarction pattern which would be recorded by a lead orientated towards the true posterior wall. The tall R wave is the mirror-image of the pathologic Q wave (Fig. 40), the depressed S-T segment is the mirror-image of the elevated S-T segment, and the tall, symmetrical T wave is the mirror-image of the deeply inverted T wave (dotted line in Diagram B of Fig. 38).

THE PHASE OF RESOLUTION

Resolution of the electrocardiographic infarction pattern progresses from the fully evolved phase (illustrated in Fig. 41). During the few weeks after the fully evolved phase, there is a gradual return of the elevated S-T segments to the baseline. Concomitantly, *tall symmetrical T waves* appear in leads orientated to the *uninjured surface* illustrated by Diagram 2 of Fig. 41 and Fig. 42). The abnormal T waves gradually return to a normal or near-normal configuration (illustrated by Diagram 3 of Fig. 41). The pattern then stabilizes into a residual state where the only evidence of a previous myocardial infarction may be an abnormal Q wave in leads orientated to the infarct scar (illustrated by Diagram 4 of Fig. 41; and Fig. 43). It must be emphasized, however, that the S-T segment and T wave usually reflect the stigmata

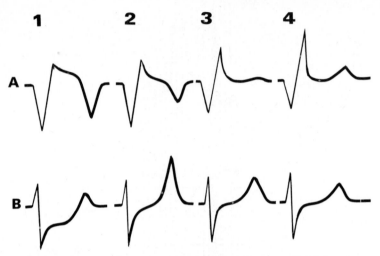

FIG. 41. Diagrams illustrating the resolution of myocardial infarction.
(A) Lead orientated to the injured surface. (B) Lead orientated to the
uninjured surface.

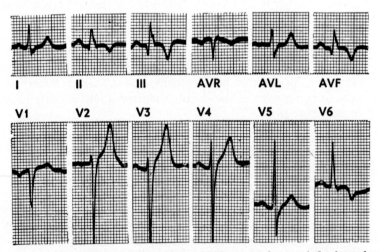

FIG. 42. Electrocardiogram showing the features of recent inferolateral
myocardial infarction. Note the Q wave, coved S-T segment and acutely
inverted T wave in Standard leads II and III and lead AVF; lead V6
shows a coved S-T segment with inverted T wave indicating lateral
extension of the infarct. The coved S-T segments are not elevated and
tall symmetrical T waves are present in leads V2 to V4 indicating that
the infarct is probably about 2 weeks old.

of coronary insufficiency, e.g. horizontality of the S-T segment, symmetry of the T wave (see page 39).

It will therefore be evident that the acuteness of a myocardial infarction is diagnosed electrocardiographically primarily by the behaviour of the S-T segment and the T wave. Thus:

ACUTE INFARCTION

Hyperacute phase: Slope-elevation of the S-T segment
                       Tall widened T wave
                       Increased ventricular activation time
Fully evolved phase: Pathological Q wave
                       Coved and elevated S-T segment
                       Inverted symmetrical T wave

OLD INFARCTION

Pathological Q wave
S-T segments and T waves which may be normal, equivocal or diagnostic of coronary insufficiency.

VENTRICULAR ANEURYSM

Note: The persistence of the typical infarction pattern—Q wave, raised S-T segment and inverted T wave—for 6 months or longer after the acute attack, suggests the development of a **ventricular aneurysm**.

EVALUATION OF Q WAVE SIGNIFICANCE IN MYOCARDIAL INFARCTION

The following factors must be taken into consideration in the assessment of Q wave significance:

(a) The specific leads in which the Q waves appear.
(b) The number of leads in which the Q waves appear.
(c) The width and depth of the Q wave.
(d) The presence of associated bundle branch block.
(e) Collateral electrocardiographic evidence of coronary artery disease.

Normal Q waves

Small q waves are normally present with normal intraventricular conduction in (a) the left precordial leads, lead AVL and Standard lead I with a horizontal heart position or left axis deviation; (b) in Standard leads II, III and lead AVF with a vertical heart position or right axis deviation. These small q waves are but a reflection of normal septal activation.

Deep wide Q waves or QS complexes are normally present in lead

AVR, and may possibly also be present in lead V1. This is due to the fact that the positive poles of these leads are orientated towards the cavity or the basal regions of the heart, so that the activation process moves away from these leads (see page 102).

Pathological Q waves
Pathological Q waves have the following characteristics:

(a) The Q wave is **wide**, 0.04 sec in duration or longer.
(b) The Q wave is **deep**, usually greater than 4 mm in depth.
(c) The Q wave is usually associated with a **substantial loss in the height of the ensuing R wave**. A rough but not invariably accurate guide is a Q wave whose depth is more than 25 per cent the height of the ensuing R wave.
(d) The aforementioned pathological Q wave characteristics must appear in leads which do not normally have deep and wide Q waves, i.e. they have no significance of infarction when they appear in leads AVR and possibly lead V1 (see above).
(e) **Pathological Q waves are usually present in several leads**, e.g. with inferior infarction, Q waves will be present in Standard leads II, III and lead AVF; with anterolateral infarction, pathological Q waves will be present in Standard lead AVL and the lateral precordial leads—leads V5 and V6.

Q waves and bundle branch block
In the presence of *right bundle branch block*, q or Q waves generally have the same significance as when they are associated with normal intraventricular conduction (see page 62).

In the presence of *left bundle branch block*, the normal septal q waves disappear from leads orientated to the left ventricle—usually leads V5 and V6. Thus, in the presence of left bundle branch block, the manifestation in these leads of any small initial q wave—no matter how small—is therefore pathological, and usually signifies myocardial infarction; an infarction that usually involves the interventricular septum.

Furthermore, in left bundle branch block, Q waves or QS complexes which resemble the pathological Q waves of myocardial infarction may appear in leads orientated to the right ventricle—particularly lead V1. This is an effect of the left bundle branch block and does not signify infarction.

THE SIGNIFICANCE OF A Q WAVE IN STANDARD LEAD III

A Q wave in Standard lead III (associated with a normal S-T segment and T wave) may be the result of an **old** inferior infarction. However, a

Q wave in this lead may frequently be present normally, and it may also occur in pathological conditions other than myocardial infarction, e.g. in acute pulmonary embolism and left posterior hemiblock. Thus, the criteria of a Q wave in Standard lead III that is suggestive or diagnostic of an old inferior infarction requires further clarification.

A Q wave in Standard lead III is suggestive of an old inferior infarction when the following criteria are satisfied:

1. The duration of the Q wave must be at least 0.04 sec, i.e. one small square in width.
2. A Q wave of at least 0.02 sec in duration, i.e. half a small square in width, must be present in lead AVF.
3. A q or Q wave of any duration must be present in Standard lead II.
4. The associated R wave in Standard lead III must be at least 5 mm in height, unless the Q wave in that lead is greater than 2.5 mm.
5. The P wave in Standard lead III must be upright. This is necessary to exclude some forms of A-V nodal rhythm where an inverted P wave associated with a short P–R interval may mimic a Q wave (see Chapter 12).

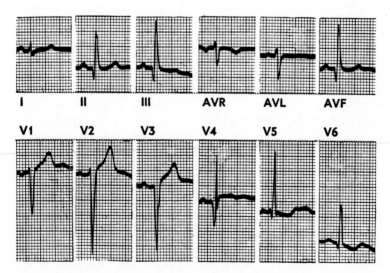

FIG. 43. Electrocardiogram showing the features of old inferior and anterolateral myocardial infarctions. Pathological Q waves are present in Standard leads II and III and lead AVF (inferior infarction), and leads V4 to V6 (anterolateral infarction). The Q waves are not associated with coved and elevated S-T segments, or acutely inverted T waves, thus indicating old infarction. Note the 'mirror-image correction mark' shape of the S-T segments in leads V5 and V6 due to digitalis effect.

Note: A negative delta wave in the W-P-W syndrome may also mimic a pathological Q wave (see Chapter 19, Figs. 191 and 192).

A normal q wave in Standard lead III frequently disappears on deep inspiration; this should be a routine procedure when recording Standard lead III.

See also the vectorial concept of Q wave significance in Standard lead III (page 111).

THE ELECTROCARDIOGRAM AS A PROGNOSTIC GUIDE IN MYOCARDIAL INFARCTION

The following electrocardiographic features are usually, but not invariably, associated with a relatively adverse prognosis in acute myocardial infarction:

1. **Extensive infarction:** The infarction pattern is seen in many leads, e.g. (a) *extensive* anterior infarction—the infarction pattern is seen in leads V1 to V6, as well as in lead AVL and Standard lead 1; (b) inferolateral infarction with true posterior extension.
2. **Multiple infarctions:** Acute infarction associated with evidence of pre-existing old infarctions, e.g. acute anterior infarction combined with evidence of old inferior infarction.
3. **Bundle branch blocks:** The development of bundle branch connotes an adverse prognosis; left bundle branch block is a more adverse prognostic sign than right bundle branch block.
4. **Ectopic ventricular rhythms:** The following ectopic ventricular rhythms are listed in order of increasing prognostic adversity: frequent unifocal ventricular extrasystoles; unifocal ventricular estrasystoles in bigeminal rhythm; unifocal ventricular extrasystoles in pairs; multifocal ventricular extrasystoles; ventricular tachycardia (see also Fig. 146 and page 152). The manifestation of ventricular extrasystoles with a very short coupling interval—the **'R on T' phenomenon** is particularly ominous (see page 152).
5. **Atrioventricular block:** The development of atrioventricular block always worsens the prognosis; the higher the degree of block, the more adverse the prognosis (Cohen, Doctor & Pick, 1958[3]). In patients who survive the initial episode, the long-term prognosis is not affected by the persistence of atrioventricular block.

CORONARY INSUFFICIENCY

TRANSIENT MYOCARDIAL ISCHAEMIA. ANGINA PECTORIS. THE 'MINOR' SIGNS OF CORONARY ARTERY DISEASE

Coronary artery disease may be reflected by changes in the QRS complex, S-T segment, T wave and the U wave. These changes may be present at rest or they may be precipitated by methods which induce transient myocardial ischaemia, e.g. exercise.

THE ELECTROCARDIOGRAPHIC EFFECTS OF CORONARY INSUFFICIENCY

The QRS deflection represents the activation or depolarization process of the ventricles; the S-T segment and T wave represent the recovery or repolarization process of the ventricles. The effects of coronary insufficiency may be reflected in both processes. The earliest changes, however, are usually evident in repolarization, i.e. in the S-T segment and the T wave. As a rule, changes in depolarization tend to be permanent, whereas changes in repolarization tend, initially, to be temporary or evanescent.

1. THE EFFECTS ON THE QRS COMPLEX

Coronary insufficiency may cause **bundle branch block** particularly left bundle branch block (see Chapter 3), and **significant left axis deviation** (see Chapter 7).

2. THE EFFECTS ON THE S-T SEGMENT

Coronary insufficiency may **depress** and **alter the shape** of the S-T segment. It may, on occasion, also present with transient *elevation* of the S-T segment as a manifestation of the variant form of angina pectoris—Prinzmetal's Angina.

THE EFFECT ON THE SHAPE OF THE S-T SEGMENT
Normally, the S-T segment merges smoothly, gradually and imperceptibly with the ascending limb of the T wave so that a separation between the two is difficult or impossible to define (A in Fig. 44; a in Fig. 46).

One of the earliest signs of coronary insufficiency is an alteration in

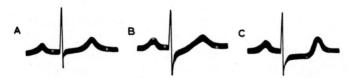

Fig. 44. Diagrammatic illustration showing (A) Normal QRST complex, (B) Junctional S-T segment depression, (C) Plane S-T segment depression.

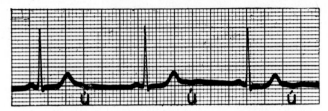

FIG. 45. Electrocardiogram—lead V5 showing signs of coronary insufficiency, viz. horizontality of the S-T segment, sharp-angled ST-T junction and inverted U wave.

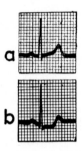

FIG. 46. Electrocardiogram—lead V5. (a) Before exercise, showing normal QRST complex. (b) After exercise, showing signs of coronary insufficiency, viz. plane depression of the S-T segment with sharp-angled ST-T junction.

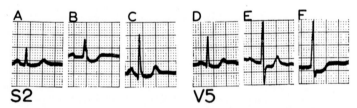

FIG. 47. Electrocardiograms—Standard lead II and lead V5—illustrating various forms of S-T segment depression. Examples A, B, C, D and F illustrate *sagging depression*. Example E illustrates plane depression; note the sharp-angled ST-T junction.

the shape of the S-T segment resulting in a **sharp-angled ST-T junction** (Figs. 45, 46 and 47E). The effect is an appearance of **horizontality** of the S-T segment. A further stage in the evolution of this effect is **depression of the S-T segment**—the depression of a horizontal S-T segment gives the appearance of **plane depression** (Fig. 44C; Fig. 46, and see below). The S-T segment may also have a **sagging depression** (Fig. 47).

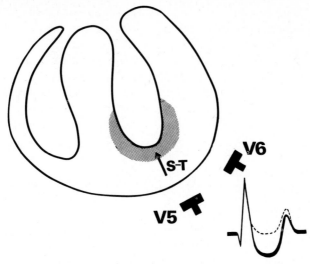

FIG. 48. Diagrammatic illustration of the subendocardial injury in angina pectoris. The transient injury results in an S-T segment shift towards the injured surface, i.e. towards the left ventricular cavity and away from leads V5 and V6; thereby resulting in S-T segment depression in these leads.

DEPRESSION OF THE S-T SEGMENT

The Mechanism of S-T Segment Depression

Transient myocardial ischaemia, as manifested clinically by the classic form of angina pectoris, results in temporary subendocardial ischaemia to the apical region of the left ventricle with transient injury to this region. The injured surface faces the left ventricular cavity (Fig. 48).

On the basis of the principles discussed earlier in this chapter, the S-T segment is deviated to the surface of injury. Thus, a lead orientated to the injured surface—in this case the left ventricular cavity—e.g. lead AVR, will reflect the pattern of injury and ischaemia, viz. a raised S-T segment and inverted T wave. Leads facing the external surface—mainly leads V5 and V6—will reflect reciprocal S-T segment depression. These changes are discussed in greater detail with reference to the exercise test (see below and Fig. 48).

THE VARIANT FORM OF ANGINA PECTORIS

(Synonyms: Prinzmetal's Angina, Atypical Angina)

As noted above (page 40), the classic form of angina pectoris is the expression of transient sub*endo*cardial injury. In contrast to this, the variant form of angina pectoris is due to transient sub*epi*cardial injury.

The condition thus manifests characteristically with transient elevation of the S-T segments in leads orientated to the injured surface (see below).

Attention was first focused on this form of angina pectoris by Prinzmetal and his associates (1959),[20] although occasional reports had appeared previously.[10] The condition is not uncommon but has been poorly documented. It is receiving increasing attention.[5]

ELECTROCARDIOGRAPHIC MANIFESTATIONS

The following electrocardiographic features appear in leads orientated to the injured surface—usually leads V4 to V6 (Fig. 49):

1. Slope-elevation of the S-T segment.
2. Tall and widened T wave.
3. Increased ventricular activation time.

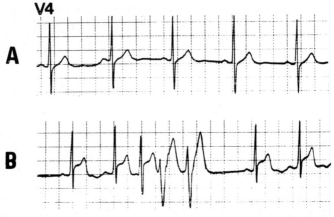

FIG. 49. Electrocardiogram A was recorded at rest and is relatively normal. Electrocardiogram B was recorded after effort and shows the manifestations of the variant form of angina pectoris: slope-elevation of the S-T segments, increased amplitude of the T waves, inverted U waves and ventricular extrasystoles.

These three manifestations constitute the classic presentation of the variant form of angina pectoris, a presentation which is, in effect, the same as that of the hyperacute phase of myocardial infarction. In the case of the variant angina pectoris, however, the manifestation is very transient, lasting but a few minutes, whereas in the hyperacute phase of myocardial infarction, the condition lasts for hours or even days. These electrocardiographic features are described in greater detail in the section on the hyperacute phase of myocardial infarction (page 21 and Diagram B of Fig. 24).

ADDITIONAL FEATURES

4. Increase in the amplitude of the R wave.
5. Diminution in the depth of the S wave of an RS complex.
6. Transient left anterior hemiblock.[2, 22]
7. Inversion of the U wave.[23]
8. Ventricular extrasystoles or even ventricular tachycardia.
9. Transient A-V block.

SIGNIFICANCE

The disorder is due to a marked narrowing of a major coronary artery.[6, 14, 15, 18, 20] The condition may also be due to marked spasm of an otherwise normal or near-normal coronary artery.[7, 32]

The variant form of angina pectoris is usually associated with a grave clinical prognosis. Infarction and/or death frequently occurs within one year of the onset.[8, 9, 17, 19, 21, 28]

3. THE EFFECTS ON THE T WAVE

The T wave is the most unstable component of the electrocardio-graphic recording. Changes of this deflection may occur with hyper-ventilation, heavy meals, anxiety, smoking, drinking iced water, changes in body position and decrease in blood pressure. Variations also occur with race and age. They are found so frequently as normal variants that when they occur as isolated phenomena their diagnostic import is uncertain.

Despite this, there are certain T wave changes that are frequently suggestive of coronary insufficiency. The T wave associated with coronary insufficiency has **symmetrical limbs** and **a sharp-pointed, arrowhead vertex** or **nadir** (Fig. 50a); the associated S-T segment usually shows an upward convexity. The T wave configuration from other causes usually shows asymmetrical limbs with a relatively blunt vertex or nadir (Fig. 50b and c).

Coronary insufficiency is also suggested when T waves in many leads are low or inverted.

Occasionally the **T wave becomes taller (as well as pointed and symmetrical)** with coronary insufficiency (Fig. 52). If, following exercise, the height of the T wave in lead V4 is 5 mm or more than the resting value, coronary insufficiency should be suspected (Lepeschkin & Surawics, 1958).[11]

THE QRS:T RELATIONSHIP

In the presence of a dominantly positive QRS deflection in Standard lead I, frank inversion of the T wave in that lead is usually abnormal.

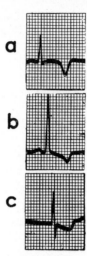

FIG. 50. Electrocardiograms (all of lead V5) showing the S-T segment and T waves changes of: (a) coronary insufficiency; (b) the 'strain' pattern usually associated with ventricular hypertrophy; (c) digitalis effect.

Furthermore, in the presence of a dominantly positive QRS deflection in Standard lead I, a **T wave in Standard lead I that is lower than a T wave in Standard lead III** is also frequently abnormal (Fig. 51). The T wave eventually becomes frankly inverted in Standard lead I and very dominantly upright in Standard lead III (Fig. 52). This phenomenon is an expression of a wide frontal plane QRS-T angle, i.e. a wide spread between the mean frontal plane QRS and T wave forces (see page 105).

A wide spread between the mean QRS and T wave forces may also be reflected by the precordial leads, i.e. the horizontal plane leads (see page 106 and Fig. 115). Empirically, this will result in a **T wave that is taller in lead V1 than in lead V6**, associated with a QRS complex that is dominant and upright in lead V6 (Fig. 52). This finding is suggestive of coronary insufficiency and may be one of its earliest signs (Weyn & Marriott, 1962[31]).

4. THE EFFECTS ON THE U WAVE

The U wave is a small rounded deflection occurring just after the T wave (Figs. 58 and 199). It is best seen in the precordial leads reflecting the transition zone—usually V2 to V4. It is normally in the same direction as the T wave. The deflection may be so small as to make accurate recognition difficult; and in the presence of a tachycardia, the U wave

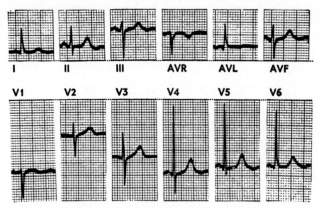

FIG. 51. Electrocardiogram illustrating the features of coronary insufficiency. Note (*a*) the T wave in Standard lead I is lower than the T wave in Standard lead III; (*b*) inversion of the U wave in Standard leads II, III, lead AVF, and leads V4 to V6; (*c*) rather horizontal S-T segments in Standard lead II and lead V6.

may be superimposed on the following P wave making recognition impossible (half-minute tracing in Fig. 54).

An inverted U wave, i.e. a U wave that is opposite in direction to the T wave, is diagnostic of cardiac disease, especially of coronary artery or hypertensive origin. When it develops after exercise it always indicates cardiac ischaemia (Figs. 49 and 54).

Note: While many of the aforementioned electrocardiographic signs are indicative, presumptive or suggestive of coronary insufficiency, it must be emphasized that the diagnosis must *not* be based on equivocal or non-pathognomonic signs, e.g. minor T wave changes, isolated T

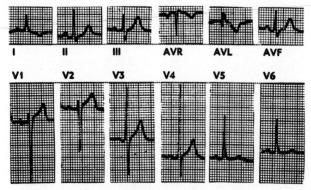

FIG. 52. Electrocardiogram illustrating the features of coronary insufficiency. Note (*a*) inversion of the T wave in Standard lead I, associated with a tall dominant T wave in Standard lead III; (*b*) the T wave in lead V1 is taller than the T wave in lead V6.

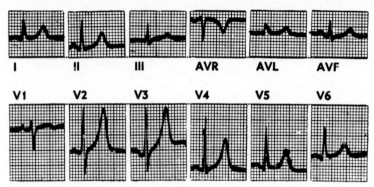

FIG. 53. Electrocardiogram showing the features of acute coronary insufficiency. Note the tall, peaked symmetrical T waves in leads V2 to V6 and in Standard leads I and II.

wave changes, junctional S-T segment depression. And it cannot be stressed too strongly that clinical judgment is paramount and that too much weight must not be placed on an equivocal electrocardiographic change as the sole criterion of coronary insufficiency.

THE EXERCISE TEST

THE PURPOSE OF THE EXERCISE TEST

A good history is usually sufficient to establish the diagnosis of angina pectoris or coronary insufficiency. At times, however, the pain is atypical and the history doubtful; objective confirmation of the diagnosis then becomes desirable. In such cases, the electrocardiographic changes seen in response to exercise may provide this confirmatory evidence, since the object of the test is to increase the demand for coronary blood flow where an inadequate flow is suspected.

THE PERFORMANCE OF THE EXERCISE TEST

The exercise test can be performed according to a standardized or a non-standardized method.

THE STANDARDIZED METHOD

Master and his associates (1942)[16] standardized the test according to sex, weight and age. Using these parameters, tables were constructed, based on the return of blood pressure and pulse rate to normal within 2 minutes. The exercise is performed on a special standardized two-step apparatus and the patient is required to do a certain number of ascents and descents in $1\frac{1}{2}$ minutes.

These principles may well be questioned, for it has not been shown that coronary artery disease, once present, runs a course which is more severe in the female; nor has it been shown that ECG changes following exercise parallel those of pulse rate and blood pressure. Furthermore, although coronary artery disease is usually more prevalent and more marked in the older age groups, it may be severe in a woman of 40 years and not at all evident in a man of 80 years.

In addition, other factors, such as emotion and training, may influence the outcome of the test and will affect any attempt to standardize it.

Nevertheless, although the validity of the exercise test as described by Master may be questioned, it should be stated that the Master two-step test is recognized in many centres and is commonly used as a routine procedure in many electrocardiographic laboratories. Provided its limitations are appreciated, it may serve a purpose as a comparative standard, e.g. (i) as a standard for insurance evaluation; (ii) as a uniform screening test in the medical examination of military and aviation personnel; (iii) as a possible research standard.

THE NON-STANDARD METHOD

Scherf recommended originally (1935)[24] and still recommends (1960),[26] that the amount of exercise the patient is required to perform be adapted to the needs of the particular individual. The patient is subjected to approximately the exertion that has been known to bring on an attack of angina pectoris. This does not mean that the patient is exercised indiscriminately until such time as he develops pain. If, for example, the patient has pain after only the slightest exertion, he may be asked to do a few knee-bends or sit up and down a few times; whereas a patient who has pain only after severe exertion may be asked to climb several flights of stairs rapidly.

If no changes are noted, and if the patient's condition warrants it, the exercise test may be repeated after a suitable interval (usually 1 hour) with a cautious increase in the amount of exercise.

The following procedures are thus recommended in the performance of the exercise test:

1. The *patient must not be in pain.* The history and physical examination must not suggest an impending myocardial infarction or acute pulmonary embolism. The patient must not be in congestive cardiac failure.
2. An electrocardiogram is recorded at rest and must be normal or at most equivocal in respect of coronary artery disease. There must be *no tachycardia.*
3. The test is preferably performed *before a meal*, since physiological

variants are more likely to occur after a meal. If the patient relates a history of angina pectoris after meals, the test should then be performed before a meal and, if negative, repeated after a meal.

4. The exercise test is performed according to the non-standardized method.

5. If pain, substernal discomfort, a feeling of faintness or pallor develop during the performance of the test, the exercise is stopped immediately. Exercise to the point of pain is hazardous and unjustifiable. *The attendance of a physician is mandatory.*

6. The electrocardiogram is recorded immediately after the exercise and at 2-minute intervals for 6 minutes, or until such time as it returns to the resting configuration.

7. The ECG changes should be observed in at least one precordial lead and one extremity or bipolar lead. S-T segment changes are usually best seen in leads with the tallest R waves—commonly leads V5 and V6, and Standard lead II; this is due to the fact that these leads are usually orientated towards the main muscle mass of the ventricles (see page 104 and Figs. 106 and 107). T wave changes that occur in Standard lead I are usually the most significant of those seen in the Standard leads.

8. The test must *not* be performed if the patient is reluctant or un-co-operative.

THE INTERPRETATION OF THE EXERCISE TEST

Certain electrocardiographic changes which follow exercise are always pathological; others, however, can only be regarded as normal physiological variants. Nevertheless, the transition between what is normal and abnormal is extremely difficult, if not impossible, to define; and there is a considerable degree of overlap between the two. Since it is never possible to rule out false negative tests, i.e. a normal ECG does not necessarily exclude coronary artery disease, it is best to establish stringent criteria of major abnormality in order to avoid labelling borderline physiological variants as abnormal. Less stringent criteria are used for insurance purposes and the screening of military and aviation personnel.

The electrocardiographic changes which follow exercise may affect all components of the record—the P wave, the P-R segment, the QRS complex, the S-T segment, the T wave and the U wave; in addition, abnormal rhythms may occur. These changes are summarized in Table I. Most of the significant changes have already been described above in the section titled 'The Electrocardiographic Effects of Coronary Insufficiency'; it must be stressed that these changes have the same significance when precipitated by exercise as when present in the 'resting' or control tracing.

CHANGES AFFECTING THE P WAVE (Table I)

Following exercise there is a tendency for *right axis deviation of the P wave,* so that the P waves tend to become taller in Standard leads II and III. These are normal physiological variants (Fig. 54).

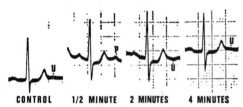

CONTROL   1/2 MINUTE   2 MINUTES   4 MINUTES

FIG. 54. Electrocardiographic recording during an exercise test. Standard lead I. *Note*: Positive U wave in the control tracing and an inverted U wave in the 2-minute tracing; superimposition of the P wave on the U wave during the tachycardia of the half-minute tracing; 1.25 mm *plane* depression of the S-T segment with *sharp-angled ST-T junction* in the half-minute and 2-minute tracings; the smooth transition of the ST-T junction in the control tracing; the downward slope of the P-R segment in the half-minute tracing. There is also a prolonged P-R interval in the control and 4-minute tracings.

Comment: The S-T segment depression, plane configuration of the S-T segment with sharp-angled ST-T junction and inverted U wave makes this test definitely positive and diagnostic of coronary insufficiency.

CHANGES AFFECTING THE P-R SEGMENT (Table I)

The *P–R interval normally shortens with exercise* (Fig. 54).

The effect on the Tp wave

Atrial depolarization is normally followed by atrial repolarization, i.e. as a T wave follows the QRS complex, so a corresponding 'T' wave normally follows the P wave. This atrial T wave is known as the Ta or Tp wave and is normally opposite in direction to the P wave. It is unusually masked by the ensuing QRST deflection and is therefore best seen following isolated P waves such as are found during A-V block (Fig. 55).

Following exercise, the Tp deflection normally becomes more pronounced and may cause the P-R segment to have a downward slope (Fig. 54, half-minute and 2-minute tracings). It may cause junctional depression of the S-T segment, thus producing a false positive S-T segment depression.

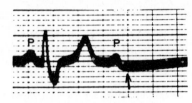

FIG. 55. Electrocardiogram showing sinus rhythm with 2:1 A-V block. The first P wave is followed by a QRS complex which masks the Tp deflection; the second P wave is not followed by a QRS complex and the Tp deflection (arrow) is thus seen as a shallow depression of 0.75 mm.

CHANGES AFFECTING THE QRS COMPLEX

(Table I; and see also section above 'The Electrocardiographic Effects of Coronary Insufficiency'.)

There is a *normal tendency for right axis deviation* of the QRS complex following exercise.

The development of abnormal widening of the QRS complex is regarded as a positive test. The appearance of **left bundle branch block** after exercise is pathological. The development of right bundle branch block is usually abnormal but may occasionally occur as a normal variant, especially when it is dependent upon critical rate (see Fig. 174, page 182). The development of left axis deviation after exercise is usually abnormal.

CHANGES AFFECTING THE S-T SEGMENT

(Table I; see also section above 'The Electrocardiographic Effects of Coronary Insufficiency'.)

Coronary insufficiency causes S-T segment depression. This is best seen in leads with the tallest R waves—usually lead V5 and Standard lead II (see page 104).

The amount of depression that is considered definitely abnormal is the most disputed point in the interpretation of the exercise test. Figures in excess of 0.5 mm (Master *et al.*, 1942[16]), 0.75 mm (Lepeschkin & Surawics, 1958[11]; Levan, 1945[12]), 1.0 mm (Unterman & de Graff, 1948[30]), 1.5 mm (Biorck, 1946[1]) and 2 mm (Scherf & Schaffer, 1952[27]) depression in the precordial leads V4 and V5 have all been considered as definitely abnormal. The matter is further complicated by the fact that it is at times difficult to judge the position of the baseline as a reference point from which to measure the depression, and the depressing effect of the Tp deflection must also be taken into account (see above). The best baseline or isoelectric level to use is the U-P segment, but this is often obscured during the teachycardia which so frequently follows exertion

(half-minute recording in Fig. 54). In such cases the baseline is measured from the junction of the P-R segment with the QRS complex.

The position was best evaluated by Scherf & Schaffer (1952)[27] who
stated that, since it is impossible to eliminate false negative tests, i.e.
since a negative result or normal electrocardiogram does not exclude
cardiac disease, it becomes imperative to avoid false positive tests,
consequent incorrect diagnoses, and possible iatrogenic disease. Thus
Scherf deliberately set extremely stringent criteria to avoid making
incorrect diagnoses; so that a positive test should be based on in-
contestable standards. The test is therefore only considered diag-
nostically positive when the S-T segment depression is 2 mm or more
in the precordial leads and 1.5 mm or more in the extremity leads.
Nevertheless, any depression of between 0.75 mm and 2 mm in the
precordial leads is usually abnormal (Fig. 54).

CHANGES AFFECTING THE T WAVE

(Table I; see section above 'The Electrocardiographic Effects of
Coronary Insufficiency'.)

CHANGES AFFECTING THE U WAVE

(Table I; see section above, 'The Electrocardiographic Effects of
Coronary Insufficiency'.)

CHANGES IN RHYTHM FOLLOWING EXERCISE
(Table I)

Sinus tachycardia normally follows exercise. Exercise may occasionally
precipitate left or right bundle branch block (see above).

The presence of **multiform ventricular extrasystoles** is diagnostic of cardiac disease. When they develop in response to exercise
they constitute a positive test.

Unifocal ventricular premature beats may occasionally be found in
the normal subject. Nevertheless, their presence after exercise usually
means abnormality; especially if they occur in 'showers', if they give
rise to short runs of bigeminal rhythm, if they occur in a person over
40 years of age or if they persist for several minutes or longer.

ADDITIONAL FACTORS

THE DURATION OF ECG ABNORMALITIES
AFTER EXERCISE

Electrocardiographic changes, particularly S-T segment depression,

TABLE I. Interpretation of the electrocardiographic exercise test

Component of ECG	Abnormal	Usually abnormal	Physiologically or diagnostically uncertain
P wave			Right axis deviation (taller in Standard leads II and III)
P-R segment			Downward slope
QRS complex	Left bundle branch block	Right bundle branch block Left axis deviation	Right axis deviation
S-T segment	Depression of 2 mm or more in the precordial leads	Depression of 0.75–2 mm in the precordial leads Any degree of plane or sagging depression	Junctional depression
	Depression of 1.5 mm or more in the extremity leads	'Horizontality', Sharp-angled ST-T junction	
T wave		Inversion in Standard lead I T in Standard lead I lower than T in Standard lead III Increase in height by 5 mm or more in lead V4 Symmetrical T waves—upright or inverted	Inversion in other leads
U wave	Inversion		
Ventricular extrasystoles ...	Multifocal Post-extrasystolic T wave change Post-extrasystolic U wave change	Unifocal: In 'showers' In bigeminal rhythm In a patient over 40 years	Isolated unifocal

due to coronary insufficiency tend to last longer than those caused by physiological variants. Although there are exceptions, normal variants or false positive changes usually last less than 2 minutes, whereas pathological or true positive changes commonly last 5 minutes or longer (Lepeschkin & Surawics, 1958[11]).

A depression of about 0.75 mm in the precordial leads, which is usually, though not definitely, diagnostic of cardiac ischaemia, is considerably strengthened as a criterion of positivity when the change lasts 5 minutes or longer.

THE EFFECT OF DIGITALIS ON THE EXERCISE TEST

Digitalis may markedly influence the S-T segment (Figs. 50 and 81) and positive tests have been reported in patients taking digitalis, in whom there was no evidence of coronary artery disease (Zwillinger, 1935[33]; Liebow & Feil, 1941[13]). The exercise test cannot therefore be interpreted with confidence in the presence of digitalis effect.

HYPERTENSION AND THE EXERCISE TEST

The exercise test should be interpreted with caution when there is associated hypertension with left ventricular hypertrophy and strain, since this may, at times, mimic the effects of coronary insufficiency. Following exercise, a pattern of left ventricular hypertrophy (QRS changes only) may change to one of 'strain'—S-T segment depression with T wave inversion; U wave inversion may also occur. Such T wave change, however, usually manifests with asymmetrical limbs and the vertex is not pointed (see above and Fig. 50b).

RELATIONSHIP OF ELECTROCARDIOGRAPHIC CHANGES TO THE DEVELOPMENT OF PAIN

The appearance of abnormal electrocardiographic changes does not necessarily correlate with that of pain. Although the patient should *not* be exercised to the point of pain by intent, when pain is precipitated as a result of the exercise test, it may occur long after the appearance of abnormal changes and may disappear long before such changes have regressed.

THE 'POOR MAN'S EXERCISE TEST'

Levine has styled the chance finding of an extrasystole with **post-**

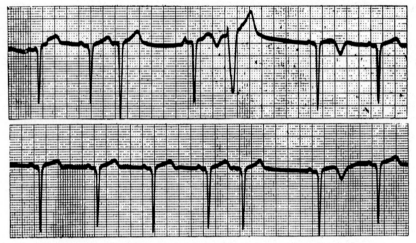

FIG. 56. Electrocardiogram (lead V1, continuous strip) showing post-extrasystolic T wave inversion. The third QRS complex in the upper strip and the fifth QRS complex in the lower strip are conducted atrial extrasystoles; the fifth QRS complex in the upper lip is a ventricular extrasystole. Note the marked inversion and symmetry of the T wave in the normal sinus complex *following* each extrasystole.

extrasystolic T wage change in the control tracing as a 'poor man's exercise test', since it gives immediate evidence of abnormality and obviates the necessity for a further, more expensive, exercise test.

The abnormality consists of a T wave change in the first *sinus* beat following an atrial or ventricular extrasystole (Figs. 56 and 57). The T wave usually becomes inverted, but may become taller than normal; any change is significant. Similar changes have been observed following blocked atrial extrasystoles (Scherf, 1944[25]) (Fig. 57). Thus, it is not the

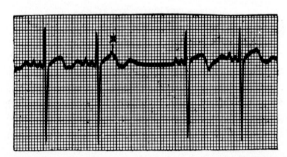

FIG. 57. Electrocardiogram (lead V3) showing a blocked atrial extrasystole with post-extrasystolic T wave inversion. The P wave of the extrasystole—labelled X—is superimposed upon the S-T segment of the second QRST complex. Note the T wave inversion in the sinus beat following the extrasystole.

extrasystole *per se* that causes this change, but rather it is the pause it occasions that evokes the change (Scherf, 1944[25]).

The U wave may also become momentarily inverted following an extrasystole—**post-extrasystolic U wave inversion** (Fig. 58).

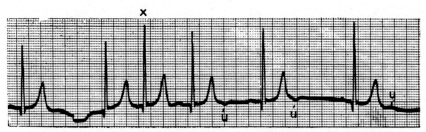

FIG. 58. Electrocardiogram (Standard lead II) showing post-extra-systolic U wave inversion. X represents an atrial extrasystole. Note the U wave inversion in the two sinus beats following the extrasystole.

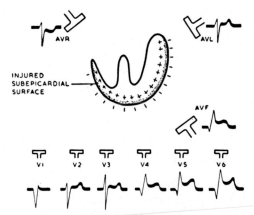

FIG. 59. Diagrammatic illustration of acute pericarditis.

PERICARDITIS

ACUTE PERICARDITIS

Acute pericarditis injures the epicardial surface of the heart. This results in a **shell of injured tissue surrounding the heart** (Fig. 59).

This injury is reflected as a raised S-T segment in leads orientated to the affected surface (refer to the beginning of this chapter for an explanation of this injury effect). As there is no myocardial ischaemia, the T waves remain upright. This results in a characteristic shape to the S-T segment, viz. it is **raised and concave upwards** (Figs. 59 and 60). This pattern is reflected in all leads facing the injured surface, i.e.

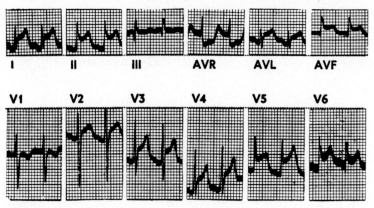

FIG. 60. Electrocardiogram of acute pericarditis. Note (*a*) the raised, concave upward S-T segment in nearly all leads, and (*b*) the sinus tachycardia.

most leads except lead AVR which faces the cavity of the heart—the uninjured surface—and thus records a depressed S-T segment, and Standard lead III which usually reflects an equiphasic S-T segment. This is because the S-T segment vector is commonly directed at $+30°$ on the frontal plane hexaxial reference system. The S-T segment vector is thus at right angles to the Standard lead III axis and parallel to the lead AVR axis. It is consequently maximal, but negative, in lead AVR.

CHRONIC PERICARDITIS. PERICARDIAL EFFUSION. CONSTRICTIVE PERICARDITIS

With resolution of the acute stage of pericarditis, the S-T segments become isoelectric. The development of pericardial effusion or constrictive pericarditis results in **generalized low voltage** and the **T waves**

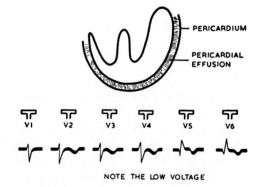

FIG. 61. Diagrammatic illustration of pericardial effusion.

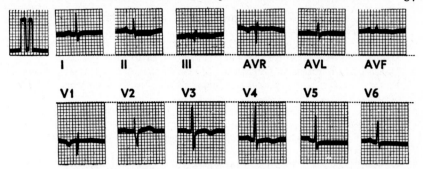

FIG. 62. Electrocardiogram showing the features of pericardial effusion. Note the generalized low voltage and the low to inverted T waves throughout. Standardization is correct, i.e. one millivolt causes a deflection of one centimetre.

become low, isoelectric or inverted in all leads orientated to the surface of the heart, i.e. most leads excepting lead AVR (Figs. 61 and 62). The low voltage is due to short-circuiting of the electrical impulse through the surrounding fluid or thickened pericardium.

Note: The same electrocardiographic pattern may be due to **myxoedema** or **hypopituitism**. (For other causes of generalized low voltage, see page 222.)

SUMMARY
> *Acute Pericarditis*
>> Normal voltage
>> Raised, concave upward S-T segments in leads orientated to the heart surface.
> *Chronic Pericarditis*
>> Generalized low voltage
>> Low to inverted T waves in leads orientated to the heart surface.

REFERENCES

1 BIORCK B. (1946) Anoxemia and exercise tests in the diagnosis of coronary diseases. *Amer. Heart J.* **32**, 689.
2 BOBBA P., VECCHIO C., DI GUGLIELMO L., SALERNO J., CASARI A. & MONTEMARTINI C. (1972) Exercise-induced RS-T elevation. Electrographic and angiographic observations. *Cardiology* **57**, 162.
3 COHEN D. B., DOCTOR, LE ROY & PICK A. (1958) The significance of atrioventricular block complicating acute myocardial infarction. *Amer. Heart J.* **2**, 215.
4 DUNN W. J., EDWARDS J. E. & PRUITT R. D. (1956) The electrocardiogram in infarction of the lateral wall of the left ventricle. *Circulation* **14**, 540.
5 EDITORIAL (1971) Atypical angina. *Brit. Med. J.* **1**, 62.
6 FORTUIN N. J. & FRIESINGER G. C. (1970) Exercise-induced S-T segment

elevation. Clinical, electrocardiographic and arteriographic studies in twelve patients. *Amer. J. Med.* **49,** 459.

7   GIANELLY R., MAGLER F. & HARRISON D. C. (1968) Prinzmetal's variant angina with only slight coronary atherosclerosis. *Calif. Med.* **108,** 129.

8   HARDEL M., BAJOLET A., GUERIN R., ELAERTS J. & GERARD J. (1969) Angor de Prinzmetal. A propos d'un cas complique d'infarctus du myocarde. *Arch. Mal. Coeur* **62,** 1267.

9   JOUVE A., GUIRAN J. B., VIALLET H., GRAS A., BLANC M., ARNOUX M., ROUVIER M. & BRUNEL J. C. (1969) Les modifications electrocardiographiques au cours des crises d'angor spontane. A propos de la forme decrite par Prinzmetal. *Arch. Mal. Coeur* **62,** 331.

10   KROOF I. G., JAFFE H. L. & MASTER A. M. (1949) The significance of RS-T elevation in acute coronary insufficiency. *Bull. NY Acad. Med.* **25,** 465.

11   LEPESCHKIN E. & SURAWICS B. (1958) Characteristics of true-positive and false-positive results of electrocardiographic Master two-step exercise tests. *New Engl. J. Med.* **258,** 511.

12   LEVAN J. B. (1945) Simple exertional electrocardiography as an aid in diagnosis of coronary insufficiency. *War Med.* **7,** 353.

13   LIEBOW I. M. & FEIL H. (1941) Digitalis and normal work electrocardiogram. *Amer. Heart J.* **22,** 683.

14   MACALPIN R. (1970) Variant angina pectoris (letter) *New Engl. J. Med.* **282,** 1491.

15   MACALPIN R. N. & KATTUS A. A. (1967) Angina pectoris at rest with preservation of exercise capacity—angina inversa. *Circulation* **35–36** (Supp. II), 176 (Abstr.).

16   MASTER A. M., FRIEDMAN R. & DACK S. (1942) The electrocardiogram after standard exercise as a functional test of the heart. *Amer. Heart J.* **24,** 777.

17   POGGI L., BORY M., PINAS E., D'JOUNO J., DJIANE P., FRANCOIS G., SERRADIMIGNI A. & AUDIER M. (1969) L'enregistrement electrographique continu dans l'angor de Prinzmetal. *Arch. Mal. Coeur* **62,** 1241.

18   PRINZMETAL M., EKMEKCI A., KENNAMER R., KWOCZYNSKI J. K., SHUBIN H. & TOYOSHIMA H. (1960) Variant form of angina pectoris; previous undelineated syndrome. *JAMA* **1,** 794.

19   PRINZMETAL M., EKMEKCI A., TOYOSHIMA H. & KWOCZYNSKI J. K. (1959) Angina pectoris. III. Demonstration of a chemical origin of S-T deviation in classic angina pectoris, its variant form, early myocardial infarction, and some non-cardiac conditions. *Amer. J. Cardiol.* **3,** 276.

20   PRINZMETAL M., KENNAMER R., MERLISS R., WADA T. & BOR N. (1959) Angina pectoris. I. A variant form of angina pectoris. *Amer. J. Med.* **27,** 374.

21   ROBINSON J. S. (1965) Prinzmetal's variant of angina pectoris. *Amer. Heart J.* **70,** 797.

22   RUSER H. R. (1970) Prinzmetalische angina pectoris. *Ztschr. Kreislaufforsch.* **9,** 849.

23   SCHAMROTH L. & LEVENSTEIN J. (1974) The electrocardiographic characteristics of the variant—Prinzmetal's—atypical form of angina pectoris manifesting in complicating ventricular extrasystoles. *S. A. Med. J.* **48,** 1146.

24   SCHERF D. (1935) Koronarerkrankungen. *Ergebn. inn. Kinderheick* **20,** 237.

25   SCHERF D. (1944) Alterations in the form of T waves with changes in heart rate. *Amer. Heart J.* **28,** 332.

26   SCHERF D. (1960) Development of the electrocardiographic exercise test. *Amer. J. Cardiol.* **5,** 433.

27   SCHERF D. & SCHAFFER A. I. (1952) The electrocardiographic exercise test. *Amer. Heart J.* **43,** 927.

28 Silverman M. E. & Flamm M. D. (1971) Variant angina pectoris. Anatomic findings and prognostic implications. *Ann. Intern. Med.* **75,** 339.

29 Tulloch J. A. (1952) The electrocardiographic features of high postero-lateral myocardial infarction. *Brit. Heart J.* **14,** 379.

30 Unterman J. B. & de Graff A. C. (1948) Effect of exercise on the electrocardiogram (Master '2-step' test) in diagnosis of coronary insufficiency. *Amer. J. med. Sci.* **215,** 671.

31 Weyn A. S. & Marriott H. J. L. (1962) The T-V1 taller than T-V6 pattern. Its potential value in the early recognition of myocardial disease. *Amer. Heart J.* **10,** 764.

32 Whiting R. B., Klein M. D. & van der Veer J. (1970) Variant angina pectoris. *New Engl. J. Med.* **282,** 709.

33 Zwillinger L. (1935) Die Digitaliseinwirkung auf das Arbeits-Elektrokardiogramm. *Med. Klin.* **30,** 977.

CHAPTER 3

Bundle Branch Block

Bundle branch block refers to a delay or block of conduction in the right or left main branches of the bundle of His.

RIGHT BUNDLE BRANCH BLOCK

In right bundle branch block the right ventricle is stimulated by the impulse from the left bundle branch which passes to the right side of the septum below the block and then to the right ventricle (Fig. 63, Vector 1). Activation of the right ventricle is thus delayed.

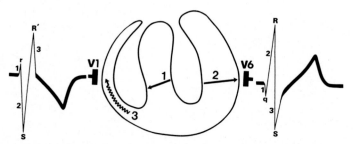

FIG. 63. Diagram illustrating ventricular depolarization in right bundle branch block, and its effect on a lead orientated to the right ventricle (lead V1) and a lead orientated to the left ventricle (lead V6).

Depolarization of the septum thus occurs normally, viz. from left to right (Vector 1 of Fig. 63). This is followed by depolarization of the free wall of the left ventricle in the usual manner, viz. from right to left (Vector 2 of Fig. 63). Finally, the free wall of the right ventricle is depolarized by an impulse from left to right (Vector 3 of Fig. 63). This force is also directed anteriorly.

This final activation of the free wall of the right ventricle is *slow* and *anomalous* in character, tending to be longitudinal or tangential rather than transverse (endocardial–epicardial). It would seem that the Purkinje system is programmed for the rapid transmission of the activation process from a central distributing point which is normally sub-endocardial. Activation entering the system from another direction, i.e. within the myocardium, is also transmitted but in a bizarre, relatively slow and ineffective manner. As a result, the deflection resulting from this form of anomalous activation is relatively increased in magnitude and slow.

SUMMARY

Sequence of depolarization:

    1. Left to right through the septum.
    2. Right to left through the free wall of the left ventricle.
    3. Left to right through the free wall of the right ventricle. This force is also directed anteriorly.

This sequence results in a widened and notched QRS complex—an **rSR or M-shaped complex, in leads orientated to the right ventricle**—usually leads V1 and V2 (Figs. 63, 64, 65, 66 and 174). The proximal limb of the M-shaped complex—the R wave—is due to the stimulus spreading *towards* the electrode through the septum (Fig. 63, arrow 1). The S wave or notch in the M-shaped complex is due to the spread of the stimulus away from the electrode as it depolarizes the free wall of the left ventricle (Fig. 63, arrow 2). The R′ deflection—the distal limb of the M-shaped complex—is due to the spread of the stimulus through the free wall of the right ventricle towards the electrode (Fig. 63, arrow 3). As right ventricular depolarization occurs late, it is unopposed by left ventricular depolarization and therefore the right ventricular force will be fairly large. Furthermore, depolarization of the free wall of the right ventricle does not necessarily proceed through the specialized conduction tissue, but through ordinary myocardial tissue (see above). This will result in a bizarre shape, and contribute to the height, of the R′ deflection.

Leads orientated to the left ventricle, usually leads V5 and V6, Standard lead I and lead AVL will show a **broad and slurred S wave** representing delayed right ventricle depolarization. This is due to the spread of the late right ventricular depolarization *away* from the electrode (Fig. 63, arrow 3; leads V4–V6 in Fig. 64).

Because of the delayed and lengthened time of depolarization, the QRS complex is widened, viz. it is longer than 0.10 sec (greater than $2\frac{1}{2}$ small squares on the graph paper).

Empirically, right bundle branch block must satisfy at least two criteria: (1) there must be an R′ deflection in lead V1; and (2) there must be a delayed S wave in Standard lead I.

The S-T segment and T wave are opposite in direction to the terminal QRS deflection (these are secondary phenomena, i.e. they occur

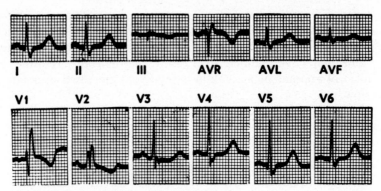

FIG. 64. Electrocardiogram showing the features of right bundle branch block. Note (*a*) the M-shaped QRS complex in the right ventricular leads—V1 and V2; and (*b*) the delayed and slurred S wave in the left ventricular leads—leads V4 to V6.

secondary to the abnormal intraventricular conduction and do not indicate primary S-T segment or T wave abnormality).

Partial right bundle branch block is diagnosed when the QRS pattern is that of right bundle branch block but the QRS complexes are not widened beyond 0.10 sec.

Note: Right bundle branch block does not alter the *initial* deflection of the QRS complex. Thus, leads orientated to the right ventricle reflect the basic rS complex—the first part of the M-shaped complex (lead V2 in Diagram A of Fig. 65). Right bundle branch block merely results in the addition of an R' deflection (lead V2 in Diagram B of Fig. 65). Leads orientated to the left ventricle reflect the normal initial qR complex (lead V6 in Diagram A of Fig. 65).

Right bundle branch block merely results in the addition of a terminal slurred S wave (lead V6 in Diagram B of Fig. 65). The initial deflection of the QRS complex in right bundle branch block therefore reflects the form of intraventricular conduction before the advent of the right bundle branch block; abnormalities in the initial deflection of the QRS complex, e.g. those due to infarction or hypertrophy will therefore still be reflected in the presence of the complicating right bundle branch block. This principle is illustrated in Diagrams C and D of Fig. 65. Diagram C illustrates the pathological Q wave of myocardial infarction in leads V2 and V6. Diagram D illustrates the anterior infarction complicated by right bundle branch block.

Note: The initial part of the QRS complex is the same as in Diagram C, the only alteration is the addition of an R' deflection in lead V2 and a slurred S wave in lead V6. A representative example of myocardial

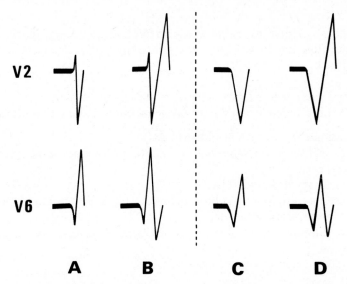

FIG. 65. Diagram illustrating the effect of right bundle branch block on the basic QRS pattern. Diagram A illustrates normal intraventricular conduction. Diagram B illustrates right bundle branch block. Diagram C illustrates myocardial infarction. Diagram D illustrates myocardial infarction complicated by right bundle branch block (see text).

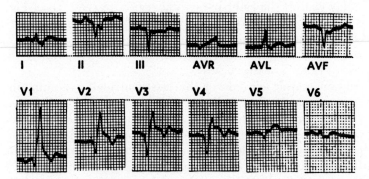

FIG. 66. Electrocardiogram illustrating acute anteroseptal myocardial infarction complicated by right bundle branch block. Note (a) pathological Q waves in leads V2 to V5; (b) the terminal R′ deflection in these leads; the R′ deflection does not mask the pathological Q waves; (c) the raised coved S-T segment in Standard lead I, lead AVL and leads V2 to V5.

infarction complicated by right bundle branch block is illustrated in Fig. 66.

Note: These principles do *not* apply to left bundle branch block, for in this condition the initial QRS forces are markedly altered as a result of the block.

SIGNIFICANCE OF RIGHT BUNDLE BRANCH BLOCK

Right bundle branch block may occur in the following conditions:

1. Occasionally, in normal individuals.
2. As a transient phenomenon in acute pulmonary embolism (see Chapter 4).
3. In coronary artery disease.
4. Partial or complete right bundle branch block is found in 95 per cent of cases of atrial septal defect.
5. As a manifestation of right ventricular diastolic overload (see Chapter 4).
6. In active carditis, e.g. diphtheritic.

LEFT BUNDLE BRANCH BLOCK

In left bundle branch block, the left ventricle is activated by the impulse from the right bundle branch which passes to the left side of the septum below the block (Vector 1a in Fig. 67). This activation process is complemented or reinforced by some activation of the free right ventricular wall in the right paraseptal region (Vector 1b of Fig. 67). This is followed by the activation process of the free wall of the right ventricle—a vector of small magnitude (Vector 2 of Fig. 67). This, in turn, is followed by the delayed activation of the free wall of the left ventricle (Vector 3 of Fig. 67).

Activation of the left side of the interventricular septum, the left septal mass, and the free wall of the left ventricle is *delayed* and *anomalous* in character. The anomalous activation process is an expression of slow, abnormal intramyocardial conduction. It has been shown that the Purkinje system is in fact used in this anomalous form of left bundle branch block activation, but the activation process tends to be longitudinal, tangential or oblique, rather than centrifugal (an endocardial to epicardial spread). It would seem that the Purkinje system is programmed for the rapid transmission of the activation process from a central distributing point which is normally the left ventricular subendocardium. Activation entering the system from another direction, i.e. from *within* the myocardium, is also transmitted, but not in a very effective manner.

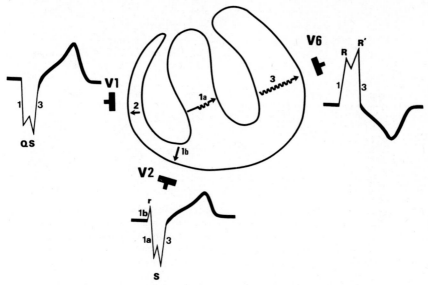

FIG. 67. Diagram illustrating ventricular depolarization in left bundle branch block, and its effect on a lead orientated to the right ventricle (lead V1), a lead orientated to the left ventricle (lead V6), and a lead orientated to the right paraseptal region (lead V2).

ELECTROCARDIOGRAPHIC MANIFESTATIONS

1. *Prolonged QRS duration*

   The QRS complex is prolonged to 0.12 sec or more, and may be as long as 0.20 sec. This is due to the delayed and anomalous activation of the left septal mass and the free wall of the left ventricle.

2. *Effect on a lead orientated to the left ventricle*

   Leads orientated to the left ventricle—usually leads V5, V6, AVL and Standard lead I—will reflect a wide, notched, *M- or plateau-shaped QRS complex* (Fig. 68). The proximal limb of the M-shaped complex results from the spread of the activation front towards the electrode, through the interventricular septum. The distal limb of the M-shaped complex is due to the spread of the activation front towards the electrode through the free wall of the left ventricle.

3. *Effect on a lead orientated to the right ventricle*

   The activation sequence will result in a wide and notched QS complex in a lead orientated to the right ventricle—lead V1 (Figs. 67 and 68). The proximal limb of the QRS complex is due to the spread of the activation front away from the electrode through the inter-

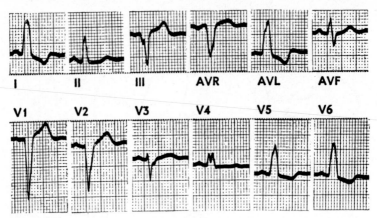

FIG. 68. Electrocardiogram showing the features of left bundle branch block. Note (a) the M-shaped QRS complex in left ventricular leads—well seen in lead V4 but barely discernible in leads V5 and V6; and (b) the broad QS complex in the right ventricular leads—leads V1 and V2. The QRS duration is 0.12 sec (three small squares).

ventricular septum. The distal limb of the QRS complex is due to the spread of the activation front away from the electrode through the free wall of the left ventricle.

4. *Effect on a lead orientated to the right paraseptal region*
   Leads orientated to the right paraseptal region—lead V2 and possibly lead V3—will reflect a small initial r wave followed by a deep, wide and notched S wave (Figs. 67 and 68). The initial r wave is due to the spread of the activation front through the right paraseptal region towards the electrode (Fig. 67). The deep, wide and notched S wave is due to the spread of the activation process away from the electrode through the interventricular septum and the free wall of the left ventricle.

5. *Secondary S-T segment and T wave changes*
   The S-T segment and T wave are opposite in direction to the terminal QRS deflection—these are secondary phenomena, i.e. they occur secondarily to the abnormal intraventricular conduction and do not indicate primary S-T segment and T wave abnormality. Thus, in leads orientated to the left ventricle (leads V5 and V6) the S-T segment is depressed and often minimally convex-upward. The T wave is inverted with a blunt nadir (Figs. 67 and 68). In leads orientated to the right ventricle (leads V1 and V2) the S-T segment is elevated and often minimally concave-upward. The T wave is upright with a relatively blunt apex (Figs. 67 and 68).

SIGNIFICANCE OF COMPLETE LEFT BUNDLE BRANCH BLOCK

Complete left bundle branch block indicates *organic heart disease*. It is commonly associated with ischaemic and hypertensive heart disease.

ARBORIZATION BLOCK

Note: When bundle branch block (right or left) is associated with low amplitude complexes, the condition is sometimes referred to as **arborization block**; this form of bundle branch block has been incorrectly attributed to a block of the Purkinje fibres.

CHAPTER 4

Ventricular Hypertrophy

LEFT VENTRICULAR HYPERTROPHY

The R wave of the qR complex recorded by a lead orientated to the left ventricle, and the S wave of the rS complex recorded by a lead orientated to the right ventricle, may indirectly be regarded as reflections of left ventricular depolarization (see Chapter 1; Fig. 8). In left ventricular hypertrophy these waves are exaggerated because of the increased electrical forces generated by the hypertrophied wall. Thus, **leads orientated to the left ventricle—usually leads V5 and V6, Standard lead I and lead AVL—will record tall R waves, and leads orientated to the right ventricle—V1 and V2—will record deep S waves** (Fig. 69).

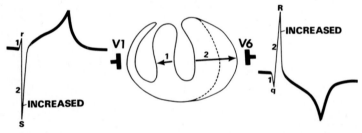

FIG. 69. Diagram illustrating the effect of left ventricular hypertrophy on a lead orientated to the right ventricle (lead V1), and a lead orientated to the left ventricle (lead V6).

If, in the adult, the sum of the S wave in lead V1 and the R wave in lead V6 exceeds 37 mm, the presence of left ventricular hypertrophy may usually be inferred, although these criteria may be normal in a thin-chested individual.

In left ventricular hypertrophy depolarization of the left ventricular wall takes longer than normal. There is thus a **delay in the onset of the intrinsicoid deflection**, i.e. the time from the beginning of the QRS complex to the apex of the R wave (measured 'horizontally') is greater than 0.045 sec (Figs. 199, 70 and 71).

Leads orientated to the left ventricle may also reflect a **'strain'**

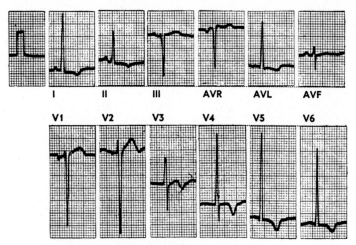

FIG. 70. Electrocardiogram showing the features of left ventricular hypertrophy and strain or left ventricular systolic overload. Note (*a*) the deep S waves in right ventricular leads—leads V1 and V2, and the tall R waves in left ventricular leads—leads V4 to V6; (*b*) the 'strain' pattern—depressed convex-upward S-T segment with inverted T wave —in left ventricular leads—leads V4 to V6; (*c*) the horizontal heart position—a qR complex in lead AVL; (*d*) the counter-clockwise rotation—rS complexes in leads V1 and V2, and qR complexes in leads V4 to V6; the transition zone is marked by the transition complex in lead V3; (*e*) the ventricular activation time as measured, for example, in lead AVL is 0.05 sec.

pattern—a depressed convex-upwards S-T segment and an inverted T wave (Figs. 69 and 70; see also Fig. 50) (see also section on left ventricular systolic overload, page 77). 'Strain' is a useful non-specific term signifying an abnormal state of the myocardium. It is possibly due to increased tension within the myocardium, or a result of the relative ischaemia resulting from the disproportion between the muscle mass and the available blood supply.

Left ventricular hypertrophy usually results in counter-clockwise rotation, and, when of long-standing duration, is often associated with a horizontal heart or left axis deviation (Fig. 71).

It must, however, be emphasized that left axis deviation is not synonymous with left ventricular hypertrophy. If, indeed, left axis deviation is associated with left ventricular hypertrophy, it reflects a complicating intraventricular conduction defect. This is due to concomitant fibrosis— the result of long-standing hypertension—which interrupts the antero-superior division of the left main bundle branch (see page 100). See Chapter 7 on the Electrical axis and also section on the Overload Concept (below).

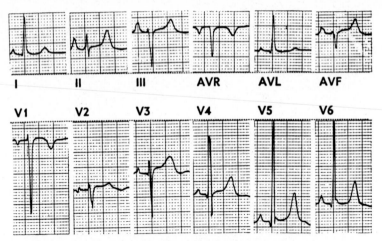

FIG. 71. Electrocardiogram showing the features of left ventricular hypertrophy with left ventricular diastolic overload. Note (*a*) the deep S wave in lead V1 and the tall R waves in leads V5 and V6; (*b*) the tall symmetrical T waves and slightly elevated concave-upward S-T segments in leads V5 and V6; (*c*) the well-marked q wave in leads V4 to V6 (compare with the q wave left ventricular systolic overload—Fig. 70); (*d*) the horizontal heart position—qR complex in lead AVL, and the counter-clockwise rotation—qR complexes in leads V4 to V6; the delay in the intrinsicoid deflection—ventricular activation time, measured in left ventricular leads, is 0.05 sec.

SUMMARY OF POSSIBLE ELECTROCARDIOGRAPHIC FINDINGS IN LEFT VENTRICULAR HYPERTROPHY

1. **Tall R waves** in leads V5 and V6, Standard lead I and lead AVL **Deep S waves** in leads V1 and V2.
2. **Delay in the onset of the intrinsicoid deflection.**
3. The **'Strain' pattern**—depressed, convex upward, S-T segment with inverted T wave in leads V5 and V6, Standard lead I and lead AVL.
4. **Counter-clockwise** rotation.
5. **Left axis deviation.**

RIGHT VENTRICULAR HYPERTROPHY

In right ventricular hypertrophy the dominant right ventricle occupies the whole anterior surface of the heart resulting in **clockwise rotation**. The heart has a **vertical position** and there is **right axis deviation** (Fig. 73).

Normally, depolarization of the interventricular septum occurs first and is followed by depolarization of the free walls of both ventricles

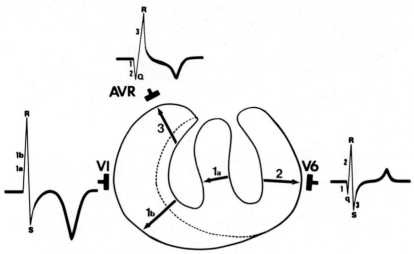

FIG. 72. Diagram illustrating the effect of right ventricular hypertrophy of leads V1, V6 and AVR.

(Figs. 6 and 7). The greater force of the left free wall counteracts the weaker force of the right free wall (Fig. 8). In right ventricular hypertrophy the potential force of the right ventricle—particularly the crista supraventricularis—is greatly increased and may even exceed that of the left free wall (Fig. 72). The R wave in right ventricular leads (V1 to V4) may thus represent both septal and right ventricular depolarization (Vectors 1a and 1b of Fig. 72) and, consequently, is increased in amplitude. The tall R wave in lead V1 may, in addition, have a small initial slur (Fig. 198).

Leads facing the right ventricle may also record a 'strain' pattern—a depressed convex-upward S-T segment with an inverted T wave (Figs. 72 and 73) (see also section on Right Ventricular Systolic Overload, page 78).

An S wave may be conspicuous in left ventricular leads due to late depolarization of a remote region of the right ventricle (Fig. 72). This force flows directly towards lead AVR—the right shoulder lead—and contributes towards a large R wave in that lead. It is also directed towards the negative poles of Standard leads I, II and III, and therefore inscribes an S wave in all three leads—this is termed the **S1, S2, S3 syndrome**. It probably reflects activation of the muscle in the right ventricular outflow tract—the **crista supraventricularis** (see also page 114).

Recent work has indicated that electrical activity in the crista supraventricularis adds greatly to the increased right ventricular forces and may even be the dominant contributing factor.

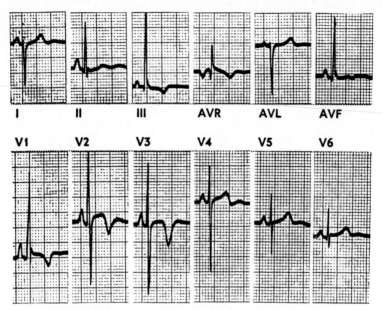

I   II   III   AVR   AVL   AVF

V1   V2   V3   V4   V5   V6

Fig. 73. Electrocardiogram showing the features of right ventricular hypertrophy and strain—right ventricular systolic overload; from a patient with the tetralogy of Fallot. Note (a) the tall R waves and 'strain' pattern in right ventricular leads—leads V1 to V4; (b) the vertical heart position—qR complex in lead AVF—and the clockwise rotation—RS or rS complexes in leads V1 to V5; (c) the tall peaked P waves—**P. congenitale**—in Standard lead II and lead V1.

SUMMARY OF POSSIBLE ELECTROCARDIOGRAPHIC FINDINGS IN RIGHT VENTRICULAR HYPERTROPHY

1. **Clockwise** rotation and **vertical** heart position.
2. **Right axis deviation.**
3. **Tall R waves** in **right ventricular leads.**
4. Small initial slur, notch or q wave in lead V1 (Fig. 198).
5. **'Strain'** pattern in **right ventricular leads.**
6. Tall R wave lead AVR.
7. The S1, S2, S3 syndrome.
   See also section on the Overload Concept (below).

THE ELECTROCARDIOGRAPHIC MANIFESTATIONS OF RIGHT VENTRICULAR HYPERTROPHY IN VARIOUS CLINICAL CONDITIONS

ACUTE COR PULMONALE

Acute cor pulmonale—due, for example, to pulmonary embolism or severe pneumonia—may manifest as follows:

Transient:

1. **Right axis deviation** (Fig. 74).
2. **Right ventricular hypertrophy and 'strain'** (as described above). This is uncommon.
3. **Right bundle branch block** (Fig. 75).
4. The **S1, Q3, T3 pattern**—prominent S wave in Standard lead I, prominent Q wave and inverted T wave in Standard lead III (Fig. 74)—usually associated with inverted T waves over the right precordium—leads V1 to V3; these inverted T waves may resemble a 'strain' or even an 'infarction' pattern.
5. **P. pulmonale.**
6. **Sinus tachycardia.**

Note: When the electrocardiogram suggests the combination of inferior and anteroseptal infarctions (Fig. 75) the possibility of acute pulmonary embolism suggests itself and must be excluded.

DIFFERENTIAL DIAGNOSIS OF ACUTE PULMONARY EMBOLISM
AND MYOCARDIAL INFARCTION

Acute Pulmonary Embolism
Changes transient—often a few hours only
Q wave in Standard lead II, insignificant, absent or rare
Injury—'Infarction'—pattern—covered, raised, S-T segment—in leads
V1–V3, i.e. it is uncommon in leads V4, V5 and V6
Always associated with sinus tachycardia.

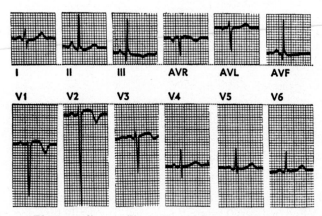

FIG. 74. Electrocardiogram illustrating the features of acute pulmonary embolism. Note (*a*) the S1, Q3, T3 pattern; (*b*) T wave inversion and slightly raised convex-upward S-T segments in leads V1 and V2; (*c*) the mean frontal plane QRS axis of +90°.

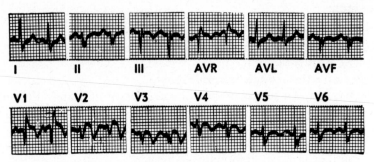

FIG. 75. Electrocardiogram showing the features of acute pulmonary embolism (autopsy revealed a pulmonary embolus in the left main pulmonary artery). Note (*a*) partial right bundle branch block—rR′ pattern in lead V1 and delayed S wave in leads V4 to V6; (*b*) the injury pattern—elevated coved S-T segments in leads V1 and V2, and to a lesser extent in leads AVF, V3, V4 and Standard lead III; (*c*) the inverted T waves in Standard lead III and leads AVF and V1 to V6; (*d*) sinus tachycardia.

Inferior Myocardial Infarction
Changes last for many days or weeks
Q wave present in Standard lead II and lead AVF.

Anteroseptal Myocardial Infarction
Infarction pattern always extends beyond lead V3, i.e. usually from leads V1–V5.

Infarction may be associated with sinus tachycardia or sinus brady-cardia or a normal sinus rhythm.

CHRONIC COR PULMONALE—EMPHYSEMA
The electrocardiographic changes of chronic cor pulmonale—emphysema (Fig. 77) are due to:

1. Right ventricular dominance.
2. The downward displacement of the heart secondary to downward displacement of the diaphragm (Fig. 76).
3. The lowered electrical transmission resulting from the surrounding voluminous lung.

This may result in:

1. P pulmonale—tall peaked P waves in Standard leads II and III and lead AVF. The frontal plane P wave axis is usually directed at +90° (see page 114).
2. A sloping P-R segment: the effect of the increased Tp deflection (see page 49).

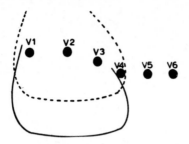

FIG. 76. Diagram illustrating the effect of the downward displacement of the heart in emphysema, i.e. the precordial electrodes become orientated to the upper or basal regions of the heart.

3. Vertical heart position, clockwise rotation and right axis deviation manifestations of right ventricle hypertrophy.
4. Low voltage; particularly in the extremity leads and leads V5 and V6: the effect of the lowered electrical transmission resulting from the surrounding emphysematous lung (Fig. 77).
5. A tendency to rS patterns with inverted T waves throughout the precordial leads (Fig. 77). This is due to the downward deplacement of the heart and diaphragm (Fig. 76). As a result, the precordial leads are orientated to the upper or basal regions of the heart which usually reflects rS patterns.

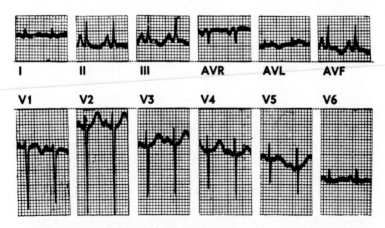

FIG. 77. Electrocardiogram showing the features of emphysema. Note (a) the tendency to low voltage in the extremity leads and leads V5 and V6; (b) the clockwise rotation—rS complexes in leads V1 to V5; (c) the tall peaked P waves—**P. pulmonale**—in lead AVF and Standard leads II and III; absence of the tall R waves in the right precordial leads which are usually associated with right ventricular hypertrophy.

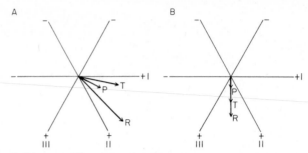

FIG. 78. Diagrams illustrating (A) Normal mean manifest frontal plane QRS, T and P wave axes, and (B) Mean manifest frontal plane QRS, T and P wave axes in emphysema.

The 'Standard lead I Sign' of Emphysema

Inspection of Standard lead I alone frequently suggests the diagnosis of emphysema, since all deflections or impressions are *minimal* and *equiphasic* on this lead (Fig. 77). This manifestation is due to the following (Fig. 78):

1. The frontal plane P wave axis in emphysema is usually directed at +90° resulting in a minimal or equiphasic deflection in Standard lead I (see Chapter 7).
2. The frontal plane QRS axis is usually directed at +90° resulting in a minimum or equiphasic deflection in Standard lead I.
3. The frontal plane T wave axis is directed either at +90° or −90° resulting in a minimal or equiphasic deflection in Standard lead I.
4. The voltage is diminished.

THE OVERLOAD CONCEPT

In the early 1950s, a concept arose attempting to correlate the various patterns of ventricular hypertrophy with cardiac haemodynamics. Cabrera & Monroy (1952)[1] indicated that ventricular hypertrophy could occur as a result of strain or overload either in systole or diastole, and this could result in different electrocardiographic manifestations. This is known as the 'overload concept'. It should be noted, however, that absolute haemodynamic-electrocardiographic correlation is by no means invariable. Indeed, the validity of the concept has been challenged. Nevertheless, the concept cannot be dismissed entirely. It forms a useful guide and requires further evaluation and clarification.

DIASTOLIC OVERLOAD

This occurs when there is an **increased flow into either ventricle**.

The overfilling of the ventricle causes an increased stretch and strain (or overload) of the myocardial fibre in diastole.

Left Ventricle Diastolic Overload occurs in:
    mitral incompetence
    aortic incompetence
    ventricular septal defect   { the left to right shunt results in an
    patent ductus arteriosus   increased return to the left ventricle

Right Ventricle Diastolic Overload occurs in:
    atrial septal defect   { the left to right shunt results in an
                             increased flow to the right ventricle
    tricuspid incompetence

SYSTOLIC OVERLOAD

This occurs when there is an **abnormal resistance to outflow** from either ventricle.

Left Ventricular Systolic Overload occurs in:
    systemic hypertension
    aortic stenosis
    coarctation of the aorta

Right Ventricular Systolic Overload occurs in:
    pulmonary hypertension
    pulmonary stenosis

ELECTROCARDIOGRAPHIC FEATURES

The diagnosis of **left** ventricular systolic and diastolic overload is made from *leads orientated to the* **left** *ventricle*, viz. leads V5 and V6, Standard

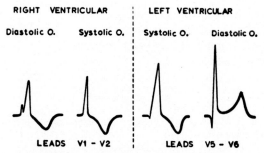

FIG. 79. Diagram illustrating the patterns of left and right ventricular systolic and diastolic overload.

lead I and lead AVL, while that of **right** ventricular systolic and diastolic overload is made from *leads orientated to the* **right** *ventricle*, viz. leads V1 and V2 (Fig. 79).

LEFT VENTRICULAR OVERLOAD PATTERNS

Left Ventricular Systolic Overload (Figs. 70 and 79)
This is characterized by:

1. Tall R waves (usually not as tall as found in left ventricular diastolic overload)
2. Delay in the onset of the intrinsicoid deflection (longer than 0.045 sec)
3. The left ventricular 'strain' pattern
   (*a*) Depressed convex-upward S-T segment
   (*b*) Inverted T waves

in leads V5 and V6, Standard lead I and lead AVL.

Left Ventricular Diastolic Overload (Figs. 71 and 79)
This is characterized by:

1. Tall R waves
2. Deep Q wave (Watson & Keith, 1962[2])
3. Tall peaked T waves
4. Slight elevation of the S-T segment

in leads V5 and V6, Standard lead I and lead ANL.

RIGHT VENTRICULAR OVERLOAD PATTERNS

Right Ventricular Diastolic Overload
This is characterized by classical right bundle branch block (Fig. 64).

Right Ventricular Systolic Overload (Fig. 73)
This is characterized by:

1. Tall R waves
2. Delay in the intrinsicoid deflection
3. Right ventricular 'strain' pattern
   (*a*) depressed convex-upward S-T segment
   (*b*) inverted T waves

in leads V1 and V2.

REFERENCES

1 CABRERA C. E. & MONROY J. R. (1952) Systolic and diastolic loading of the heart. *Amer. Heart J.* **43**, 661.
2 WATSON D. G. & KEITH J. D. (1962) The Q wave in lead V6 in heart disease of infancy and childhood, with special reference to diastolic loading. *Amer. Heart J.* **63**, 629.

CHAPTER 5

Drug and Electrolyte Effect

DIGITALIS EFFECT

Digitalis **shortens the Q–T interval** and consequently alters the S-T segment in a characteristic manner. The **S-T segment is depressed** with a straight, gradual, downward slope ending in a terminal rise to the isoelectric level; it may be likened to the **mirror-image of a correction or check mark** (Figs. 43 and 80).

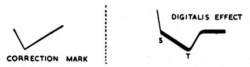

Fig. 80. Diagram illustrating digitalis effect on the S-T segment, viz. a gradual downward slope with a sharp terminal rise—the mirror-image of a correction mark.

This effect is usually seen in leads with the tallest R wave, viz. leads reflecting the dominant ventricle—leads V4 to V6 in left ventricular hypertrophy, and leads V1 to V3 in right ventricular hypertrophy. This effect suggests digitalis administration and does not necessarily indicate digitalis intoxication. When the characteristic S-T segment change appears in nearly all leads, i.e. in leads without tall R waves (leads recording rS complexes) as well as leads with tall R waves, the tracing is suggestive of digitalis toxicity. This is usually a late sign of digitalis toxicity.

Effect of digitalis on basic normal and basic abnormal S-T segments and T waves

If the S-T segment and T wave are normal or relatively normal *before* the administration of digitalis, the sharp terminal rise of the distal limb of the T wave will rise *above* the baseline following the administration of digitalis (A of Fig. 81). In the case of pre-existing abnormal S-T segments or T waves, however (i.e. low to inverted T waves associated with depressed S-T segments), the distal limb of the T wave will *not* rise

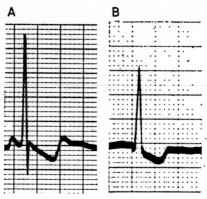

Fig. 81. (A) Lead V5. QRST complex illustrating digitalis *effect*. Note the gradual downward slope of the S-T segment and the sharp upward terminal deflection of the T wave which rises above the baseline. (B) Lead V5. QRST complex illustrating digitalis effect superimposed on pre-existing T wave abnormality. Note the terminal limb of the T wave does *not* rise above the baseline.

above the baseline (B of Fig. 81). See also effects of digitalis on the QRS-T angle (page 105).

THE DISORDERS OF CARDIAC RHYTHM ASSOCIATED WITH DIGITALIS ADMINISTRATION

Digitalis administration may be associated with any arrhythmia except the Type II (Mobitz Type II) second degree A-V block. Some typical examples are listed below and described in detail in Chapters 10 to 17.

The commonest manifestations of digitalis toxicity are (1) **bigeminal rhythm due to alternate ventricular extrasystoles**, and (2) **paroxysmal atrial tachycardia with irregular Type I second degree A-V block**.

Digitalis effect	*Digitalis toxicity*
sinus bradycardia	ventricular extrasystoles
1st degree A-V block complicating normal sinus rhythm	atrial extrasystoles
2nd degree A-V block complicating normal sinus rhythm	paroxysmal atrial tachycardia with varying Type I 2nd degree A-V block
	multifocal ventricular extra-systoles
	paroxysmal ventricular tachy-cardia

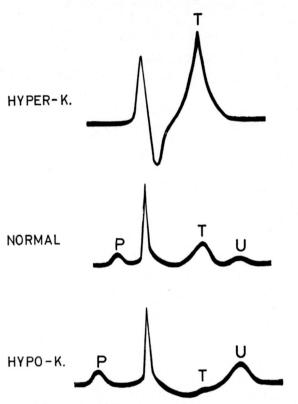

FIG. 82. Diagram illustrating the effects of hyper- and hypokalaemia.

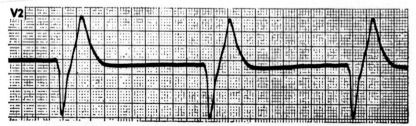

FIG. 83. The electrocardiogram (lead V2) shows: 1. A slow ventricular rhythm: rate = 28 beats per minute. 2. The features of hyperkalaemia: (a) absent P waves, (b) bizarre, low-amplitude, QRS complexes, (c) tall, wide, symmetrical T wave, (d) 'blending' of the QRS and T deflections to form large, bizarre, bi-phasic complexes.

POTASSIUM EFFECT

HYPERKALAEMIA

The following electrocardiographic sequence is associated with a progressive rise in the serum potassium level (Figs. 82 and 83).

1. The T wave becomes tall and peaked.
2. There is diminution in the amplitude of the R wave.
3. The QRS complex becomes widened.
4. The QRS complex blends with the T wave producing a wide, bizarre, diphasic deflection.
5. There is progressive diminution in the amplitude of the P wave which eventually disappears.

HYPOKALAEMIA

With a progressive diminution in the serum potassium level the following electrocardiographic sequence occurs (Figs. 82, 84 and 85):

1. The **U wave becomes prominent**.
2. The T wave becomes flattened and finally inverted. The very prominent associated U wave may thus be mistaken for a T wave,

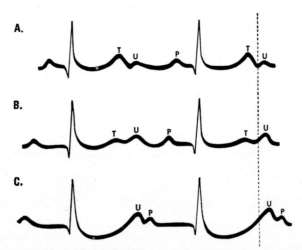

FIG. 84. Diagrams illustrating the electrocardiographic manifestation of progressive hypokalaemia. *Note*: increasing prominence of the U wave; diminishing amplitude of the T wave; increasing P–R interval; constancy of the Q–T interval (dotted line).

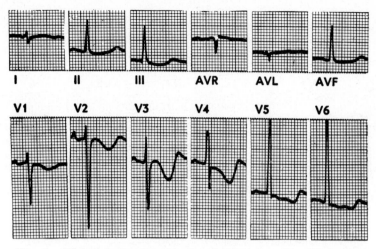

FIG. 85. Electrocardiogram showing the features of hypokalaemia. Note (a) depressed S-T segments in most leads; (b) prominent U waves in Standard leads II and III, and leads AVF and V2 to V6; the U wave, at first glance, appears to be the T wave; the T wave, however, is seen in leads V5 and V6 as a small, rounded positive deflection on the terminal part of the S-T segment; the prominent U wave, if mistaken for a T wave, gives the false impression of a prolonged Q–T interval.

and the Q–U interval may be mistaken for a prolonged Q–T interval.

3. The S-T segment becomes depressed.
4. The P–R interval becomes prolonged.
5. Rarely, there is S-A block.

CALCIUM EFFECT

HYPOCALCAEMIA

Hypocalcaemia manifests with a **prolonged Q–T interval** (Fig. 86). This is due solely to a prolongation of the S-T segment which becomes horizontal and isoelectric, 'hugging' the baseline for a relatively long period. This horizontality may mimic the horizontality of the S-T segment which is associated with coronary insufficiency (see page 40).

HYPERCALCAEMIA

Hypercalcaemia manifests with a **shortened Q–T interval**.

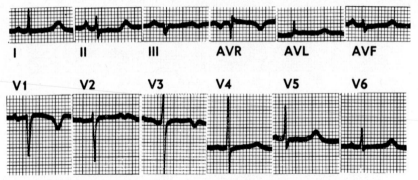

Fig. 86. The electrocardiogram was recorded from a woman with hypoparathyroidism and a low serum calcium. It shows the following features: (*a*) There is a prolonged Q–T interval. The Q–Tc was calculated to be 145 per cent. (*b*) The prolongation of the Q–T interval is due to a prolongation of the S-T segment. Note that the T wave is not particularly widened. Note, too, that the S-T segment reflects marked horizontality and is isoelectric, hugging the baseline for 6 mm, a relatively long period of 0.24 sec. There is also a tendency to a sharp angled ST-T junction.

QUINIDINE EFFECT

Quinidine has the following electrocardiographic effects:

1. **The QRS complex is widened**. If the increase in the width of the QRS complex is greater than 25 per cent of the QRS complex in the tracing recorded before quinidine administration, it reflects a toxic effect and the quinidine must be stopped.
2. **The Q–T interval is lengthened**.
3. **The T wave becomes widened, notched, and low to inverted**.

CHAPTER 6

The P Wave. Atrial Activation

The P wave reflects atrial depolarization and is recorded as soon as the impulse leaves the S-A node.

Because the S-A node is situated in the right atrium, right atrial activation begins first and is followed shortly thereafter by left atrial activation (Fig. 88). The two processes overlap, as left atrial activation begins before the end of right atrial activation.

The electrocardiographic effects of atrial activity are best seen in Standard lead II and lead V1.

ATRIAL ACTIVITY AS REFLECTED IN STANDARD LEAD II

When viewed in the frontal plane both atrial forces run roughly parallel to the Standard lead II axis (see Chapter 7 for direction of the Standard lead II axis). Both forces thus record roughly the same deflection in this lead. And since both activation processes overlap (Fig. 87), a P wave is produced that theoretically has a small notched apex. Due to the close overlap of the two forces, however, this notch is rarely seen and the P wave is consequently pyramid-shaped with a smooth, gently rounded, vertex. The amplitude in Standard lead II should not exceed 2.5 mm.

RIGHT ATRIAL ENLARGEMENT

With right atrial enlargement, the first, or right atrial component of the P wave is accentuated, resulting in a **tall P wave** with a **sharply pointed** or **peaked vertex** (Fig. 91B). This P wave is often referred to as **P. pulmonale** or **P. congenitale** for it is frequently associated with the right atrial strain that is found in pulmonary hypertension and cyanotic congenital heart disease (see also page 115).

LEFT ATRIAL ENLARGEMENT

With left atrial enlargement, the second, or left atrial component of the

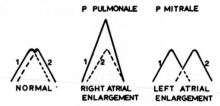

FIG. 87. Diagram illustrating the normal and abnormal components of the P wave as reflected in Standard lead II. (1) Right atrial component; (2) left atrial component.

P wave is *delayed* resulting in a **wide and notched P wave** exceeding 0.11 sec in duration (Figs. 87 and 91A). This P wave is often referred to as **P. mitrale** because of its frequent association with mitral valvular disease.

ATRIAL ACTIVITY AS REFLECTED IN LEAD V1

The right atrium is situated anteriorly in the thorax and to the right of the ventricles (Fig. 88). The left atrium is situated more posteriorly in the thorax, behind the ventricles (Fig. 88).

The right atrial force is directed towards lead V1 and thus the first, or right atrial component of the P wave is upright in lead V1 (Fig. 88A). The left atrial force is directed a little away from lead V1, and thus the second, or left atrial component is only slightly negative in this lead (Fig. 88A). As the two atrial forces overlap, the result is a P wave that is mainly upright with a slight terminal negative or equiphasic deflection (Fig. 88B).

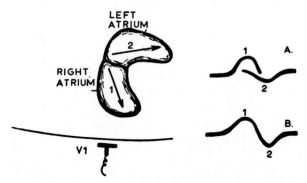

FIG. 88. Diagram illustrating the normal components of the P wave as reflected in lead V1.

RIGHT ATRIAL ENLARGEMENT

With right atrial enlargement, the right atrial component is increased, resulting in a **tall peaked P wave** (Figs. 89 and 91B) (see also page 115).

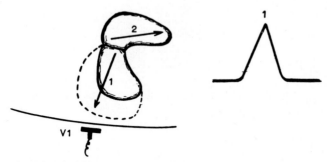

FIG. 89. Diagram illustrating the effect of right atrial enlargement on lead V1.

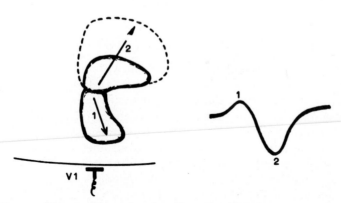

FIG. 90. Diagram illustrating the effect of atrial enlargement on lead V1.

LEFT ATRIAL ENLARGEMENT

With left atrial enlargement, the left atrial component is increased, delayed, and directed away from lead V1 (Fig. 90). The result is a **P** wave that is **mainly negative** or diphasic with an accentuated negative component (Figs. 90 and 91A).

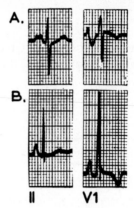

II   V1

FIG. 91. Electrocardiograms showing the features of left and right atrial enlargement. (A) Left atrial enlargement; (B) right atrial enlargement.

SUMMARY

P wave in:

	Standard lead II	Lead V1
Right atrial enlargement	Tall and peaked	Tall and peaked
Left atrial enlargement	Wide and notched	Negative or diphasic

RETROGRADE ATRIAL ACTIVATION

Retrograde activation of the atria can occur with impulses of A-V nodal and ventricular origin (see Chapters 12 and 13). Retrograde activation may also occur in certain forms of reciprocal rhythm where the sinus impulse enters an A-V nodal by-pass and returns retrograde to activate the atria a second time.

With retrograde activation of the atria, the activation front is directed cranially, i.e. away from the positive poles of Standard leads II and III, and lead AVF. These leads will consequently reflect negative P' deflections (Figs. 135, 142 and 179). The P' wave in lead V1 is usually positive and thus differs from the normal diphasic sinus P wave reflected by this lead (Fig. 181).

CHAPTER 7

The Electrical Axis

THE LEAD AXIS

Every electrocardiographic lead has a negative and a positive pole, and the location of these poles is termed the **polarity of the lead**. A hypothetical line joining the poles of a lead is known as the **axis of the lead**. Every lead axis is orientated in a certain direction depending upon the location of the positive and negative electrodes.

THE ORIENTATION OF THE LEAD AXES

The heart is situated in the centre of the electrical field which it generates. The intensity of this electrical field diminishes algebraically with the distance from its centre. Thus the electrical intensity recorded by an electrode diminishes rapidly when the electrode is moved a short distance from the heart, and less and less as the electrode is moved still further away from the heart. With distances greater than 15 cm from the heart, the decrement in the intensity of the electrical field is hardly noticeable. Consequently, all electrodes placed at a distance greater than 15 cm from the heart may, in an electrical sense, be considered to be *equidistant* from the heart. For example, an electrode placed at 25 cm from the heart will record about the same potential as one placed 35 cm from the heart.

THE STANDARD LEADS

Using this principle, Einthoven* deliberately placed the electrodes of the three Standard leads as far away from the heart as possible, i.e. on the extremities—the right arm, left arm and left leg. *These three electrodes are thus electrically equidistant from the heart.*

The leads derived from these three electrodes are conventionally as follows:

Standard lead I   Derived from electrodes on the right arm (negative pole) and left arm (positive pole) (Figs. 92 and 95).

---

* Willem Einthoven, physiologist of Leyden (1860–1927); inventor of the string galvanometer.

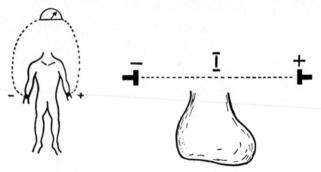

FIG. 92. Electrode placement of Standard lead I. Positive pole to left arm.

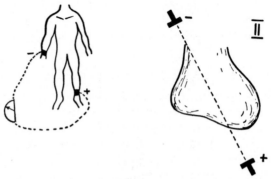

FIG. 93. Electrode placement of Standard lead II. Positive pole to left leg.

Standard lead II   Derived from electrodes on the right arm (negative pole) and left leg (positive pole) (Figs. 93 and 95).

Standard lead III   Derived from electrodes on the left arm (negative pole) and the left leg (positive pole) (Figs. 94 and 95).

The lead axes of these three leads form a triangle (Fig. 95A) and as the electrodes of these leads are regarded as equidistant from the heart, *the lead axes too may be considered to be equidistant from the heart*. These lead axes thus form an *equilateral triangle* with the heart at the centre (Fig. 95A)—the **Einthoven Triangle**.

To facilitate the graphic representation of the cardiac impulses, the three lead axes of the Einthoven Triangle may be redrawn so that they pass through the same zero point (Fig. 95B). The three lead axes thus bisect each other forming a triaxial system with each of the lead axes separated by 60° from one another.

Note: The polarity of the lead axes remains the same.

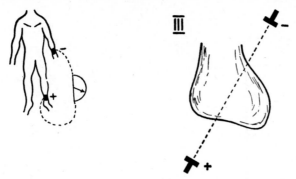

FIG. 94. Electrode placement of Standard lead III. Positive pole to left leg.

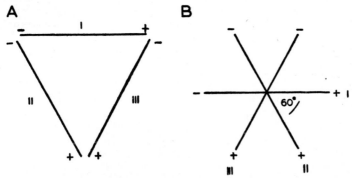

FIG. 95. (A) The Standard lead axes forming the Einthoven Triangle. (B) The lead axes of the Einthoven Triangle redrawn to form a triaxial reference system. *Note*: the direction and polarity of each lead axis remain the same.

THE UNIPOLAR LIMB HEADS

A unipolar limb lead is derived as follows: the positive pole of the lead is attached to one of the limbs, and the negative pole is attached by three wires to all three limb electrodes. The *sum* of the three limb leads is at all times equal to *zero* potential. Thus if these three leads are connected to a central terminal the potential of the terminal will be zero (see Appendix, page 234 and Figs. 212 and 213). A unipolar limb lead thus consists of a positive pole on one of the limbs and a negative pole at zero potential. Zero potential is located in the centre of the Einthoven Triangle since the centre of an equilateral triangle is equidistant from all its apices (Fig. 95A). The axis of a unipolar limb lead is therefore the hypothetical line drawn from the limb—right shoulder, left shoulder or left hip—to the centre of the Einthoven Triangle (Fig. 96A).

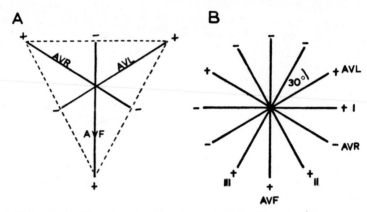

FIG. 96. (A) The triaxial reference system formed by the unipolar extremity leads. (B) The combination of the triaxial reference systems of the Standard and unipolar leads to form a hexaxial reference system.

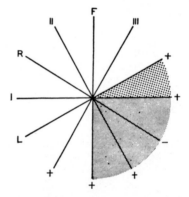

FIG. 97. The hexaxial reference system. Dark shading (0° to +90°) represents the normal range for frontal plane QRS axes. Light shading (0° to −29°) represents the equivocal range for frontal plane QRS axes.

These three unipolar lead axes also form a triaxial reference system with the axes 60° apart.

When the triaxial system of the Standard leads and the triaxial system of the unipolar limb leads are combined, they form a **hexaxial reference system** (Figs. 96A, 97 and 98). The triaxial system formed by the unipolar limb leads bisects the angles of the triaxial system formed by the Standard leads and the resulting hexaxial reference system divides the frontal plane into 30° intervals. By an irrational convention (see below), all degrees in the upper hemisphere of the hexaxial reference system are labelled negative degrees, and all degrees

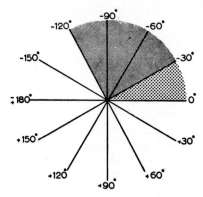

FIG. 98. The hexaxial reference system. Light shading (0° to −29°) represents the range of slight left axis deviation. Dark shading (−29° to −120°) represents the range of significant left axis deviation.

in the lower hemisphere are labelled positive degrees (Figs. 96B and 98). Thus commencing at the positive end of the Standard lead I axis (labelled 0°) and progressing counter-clockwise, the leads will be successively at −30°, −60°, −90°, −120°, −150°, −180°. Progressing clockwise, the leads will be successively at +30°, +60°, +90°, +120°, +150°, +180°.

Note: The irrational convention of labelling the hexaxial reference system as positive and negative units must not be confused with the positive and negative poles of the lead axes.

It will also be noted that, with one exception, the positive poles of the lead axes are located from −30° clockwise to +120°. The exception is the negative pole of lead AVR which is located at +30° (Figs. 96B and 97).

THE MEAN ELECTRICAL AXIS

Excitation or depolarization spreads from one region of the heart to the other in the form of an advancing wave front. This may be represented by a number of forces (Fig. 99). In Chapter 1, the electrical activity of the ventricles was, for purposes of exposition, represented in a simplified form by two forces, viz. a small initial force from left to right, followed by a larger force from right to left (Fig. 8); in reality, however, the activation process consists of a number of consecutive forces as shown in Fig. 99. The *general*, *average* or *dominant direction* of these forces is known as the *mean manifest frontal plane electrical axis* and is represented in Fig. 99 by the single force labelled M-A.

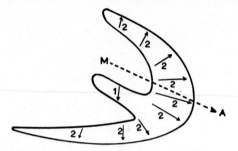

FIG. 99. Diagram illustrating depolarization of the ventricles as a series of forces or vectors. The arrow—labelled M-A—represents the mean or dominant direction of all these forces, i.e. the mean frontal plane QRS axis.

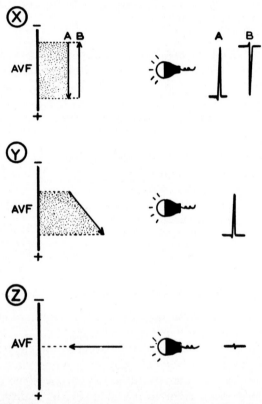

FIG. 100. Diagram illustrating the effect on a lead axis (in this case lead AVF) of forces or vectors orientated in various directions. A light source is directed at the lead axis and the imaginary 'shadow' cast by the vector on the lead axis represents the size of the deflection that will be recorded by that lead.

GRAPHING THE ELECTRICAL AXIS

If an impulse runs parallel to the axis of a lead, the force it generates will record the maximum deflection in the lead. The situation may be likened to an imaginary shadow—representing the amount of deflection—cast by the force on the lead axis (Fig. 100). If the direction of the force is towards the positive pole of the lead (A in Fig. 100 (X)) the deflection will be upwards; if the force is towards the negative pole of the lead (B in Fig. 100 (X)) the deflection will be downwards. In either case, the deflection will be maximal when compared with those recorded in other lead axes.

Such an impulse, electrical force or activation front that has both magnitude and direction is known as a *vector*.

If an impulse runs obliquely to the axis of a lead the deflection— or the shadow cast—on that lead will be less than that caused when the impulse travels parallel to the lead (Fig. 100 (Y)). The more oblique the approach to the lead, the less will be the deflection on that lead.

If the impulse runs at right angles to the axis of a lead, the deflection, or 'shadow' cast, on that lead will be nil—it is usually a small equiphasic deflection (Fig. 100 (Z)).

Note: The *nett* positive or *nett* negative deflection in any lead is gained by subtracting the smaller deflection above or below the baseline from the larger deflection above or below the baseline, e.g. the nett positive deflection in A of Fig. 100 (X) will be the tall R wave minus the small q wave.

DETERMINATION OF THE MEAN ELECTRICAL AXIS

To determine the mean frontal plane QRS electrical axis the following procedure may be adopted:

(a) **With reference to Fig. 101**

Examine the *six frontal plane leads* I, II, III, AVR, AVL, AVF. Find the lead with the *smallest* and most *equiphasic* deflection. This is lead AVL in Fig. 101. On principles enunciated above, the electrical axis must run at *right angles to lead AVL*, and it must run *parallel to Standard lead II* (refer to Fig. 100). The deflection must therefore be greatest in Standard lead II; and examination of Standard lead II confirms this. The deflection in Standard lead II is upright and the axis must therefore be directed *towards the positive pole* of that lead.

The mean electrical axis is thus located parallel to the lead axis of Standard lead II and towards its positive pole—reference to Figs. 97 and 98 shows that it is therefore located at +60°.

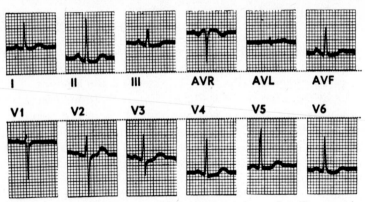

FIG. 101. Electrocardiogram: QRS axis situated at +60°; T wave axis situated at +30°; P wave axis situated at +60°.

(*b*) **With reference to Fig. 73**

The most equiphasic deflection in the six frontal plane leads is found in lead AVR. The mean manifest frontal plane axis thus runs at right angles to lead AVR. It is therefore parallel to Standard lead III and the deflection must therefore be greatest in this lead; examination of Standard lead III confirms this. The deflection is upright or positive in Standard lead III and thus the mean axis is directed towards the positive pole of Standard lead III, i.e. it is located at +120°.

However, the deflection is not absolutely equiphasic in lead AVR, i.e. it is a little more positive than negative. Thus the axis is inclined a little towards the *positive pole of lead AVR* and is therefore located at about +130°.

Similarly any electrocardiographic deflection may be expressed in terms of a mean manifest axis:

e.g. **The T Wave Axis:**
With reference to Fig. 101
1. The most equiphasic T wave deflection is found in Standard lead III.
2. The greatest T wave deflection is consequently found in lead AVR and is directed towards the negative pole of this lead.

The mean frontal plane T wave axis is thus located at +30°.

e.g. **The P Wave Axis:**
With reference to Fig. 101
1. The most equiphasic P wave deflection is found in lead AVL.
2. The greatest P wave deflection is consequently found in Standard lead II and is directed towards the positive pole of Standard lead II.

The mean frontal plane P wave axis is thus located at +60°.

The axes of some other electrocardiograms in this book are tabulated in Table II.

TABLE II. Table of electrical axes in some of the electrocardiograms in this book

| | Mean Frontal Plane Axes | | |
	QRS	T	P
Fig. 25B	+60°	−60°	+60°
Fig. 28	−50°	−40°	+60°
Fig. 32	+20°	0°	+50°
Fig. 36	−30°	−60°	+50°
Fig. 42	...	−50°	+60°
Fig. 43	+100°	+60°	+50°
Fig. 51	0°	+70°	+70°
Fig. 52	+60°	+100°	+60°
Fig. 53	+50°	+40°	...
Fig. 62	+20°	...	+50°
Fig. 70	0°	−180°	+60°
Fig. 71	−20°	+50°	+50°
Fig. 73	+130°	0°	+50°
Fig. 74	+80°	0°	+70°
Fig. 85	+90°	+120°	...
Fig. 86	0°	+30°	+60°
Fig. 101	+60°	+30°	+60°
Fig. 135	+60°	+50°	−90°

AXIS DEVIATION

The normal range for the mean frontal plane QRS axis in the adult is **0° to +90°** (Fig. 97).

RIGHT AXIS DEVIATION

Right axis deviation is diagnosed when the axis is located in the range of **+90° to +180°** (Fig. 97).

SIGNIFICANCE
Right axis deviation is usually associated with right ventricular hypertrophy. It may also be due to a left posterior hemiblock (see below).

LEFT AXIS DEVIATION

Left axis deviation is diagnosed when the axis is in the range of 0° to −120° (Fig. 98). This range may be arbitrarily sub-divided into slight left axis deviation: 0° to −29° and **significant left axis deviation: −30° to −120°.**

MECHANISM AND SIGNIFICANCE OF LEFT AXIS DEVIATION

Axes between 0° and −29° may occasionally be found in the normal subject, especially in those with obesity or a stocky build. It may also be associated with ascites or abdominal distension. In these cases the slight left axis deviation is due to a horizontal heart position. Nevertheless, axes in this zone should be viewed with suspicion as they are frequently due to organic heart disease (see below).

Axes in the region of −30° to −120°, i.e. significant left axis deviation, nearly always connote organic heart disease. Recent work (Grant, 1956[2]; Davies & Evans, 1960[1]) has shown that this condition is mainly due to **an intraventricular conduction defect involving the anterosuperior division of the left bundle branch:** a left anterior hemiblock (see below).

THE HEMIBLOCK CONCEPT

THE ANATOMY OF THE LEFT BUNDLE BRANCH SYSTEM

Shortly after leaving the main bundle of His, the left bundle branch divides into a number of rootlets which then proceed in two major

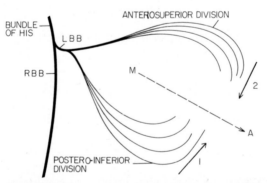

FIG. 102. Diagram illustrating the anatomy of, and conduction in, the left bundle branch. *Note*: The left bundle branch divides into two major sweeps or radiations—the anterosuperior division and the postero-inferior division. Conduction in the postero-inferior division is mainly upward and to the left; conduction in the anterosuperior division is mainly downward and to the right; simultaneous conduction through both divisions results in a mean axis—arrow labelled M-A—that is directed downward and to the left.

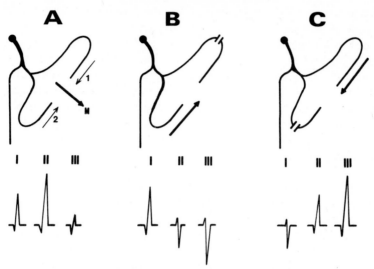

FIG. 103. Diagrams illustrating: (A) normal ventricular conduction, (B) left anterior hemiblock, and (C) left posterior hemiblock.

sweeps of radiations. These constitute the two major divisions or fascicles of the left bundle branch (Figs. 102 and 103).

The *anterosuperior division* which spreads anteriorly and superiorly over the subendocardium of the lateral wall of the left ventricle.

The *postero-inferior division* which spreads inferiorly and posteriorly over the diaphragmatic surface of the left ventricle.

The fibres of the two divisions meet and anastomose peripherally, forming a closed conduction network, a syncitium with rapid conduction properties.

The anterosuperior division of the left bundle branch is more vulnerable to disease processes than the postero-inferior division. This is because the anterosuperior division is relatively long and thin, whereas the postero-inferior division is relatively short and thick.[5] Furthermore, the postero-inferior division has a double blood supply in contrast to a single blood supply for the anterosuperior division.[6] The anterosuperior division is closer to the aortic valve, and is therefore more likely to be involved in disease processes affecting the aortic valve.[5] All these factors contribute to the greater vulnerability of the anterosuperior division.

CONDUCTION WITHIN THE LEFT BUNDLE BRANCH SYSTEM
Conduction through the anterosuperior division results in an activation front directed inferiorly and to the right (illustrated by Vector 2 in Fig. 102 and Vector 1 in Diagram A of Fig. 103). Conduction through the postero-inferior division results in an activation front directed

superiorly and to the left (illustrated by Vector 1 in Fig. 102 and Vector 2 in Diagram A of Fig. 103). Since normal activation occurs concomitantly through both divisions, the two vectorial forces summate both complementing and modifying each other's direction, and thereby resulting in a mean QRS force or vector which is directed downwards and to the left (illustrated by Vector M-A in Fig. 102 and Vector M in Diagram A of Fig. 103). This normal QRS axis is, therefore, commonly directed in the region of +60° on the frontal plane hexaxial reference system. The normal range for the mean frontal plane QRS axis in the adult is 0° to +90° (Fig. 97).

HEMIBLOCK

When conduction is delayed or interrupted in one of the divisions of the left bundle branch, it is termed a 'hemiblock'.[7]

Left anterior hemiblock

This results when conduction is interrupted in the anterosuperior division of the left bundle branch. When this occurs, the activation front of the anterosuperior division is lost, i.e. Vector 1 in Diagram B of Fig. 103 is abolished. Activation now occurs predominantly through the fibres of the postero-inferior division. And since this activation front is directed upwards and to the left, the result is a *left axis deviation* (Diagram B of Fig. 103; Diagram A of Fig. 110). The resulting mean frontal plane QRS axis is commonly in the region of −30° counter-clockwise to −90°: the region of significant left axis deviation (Fig. 98). This will manifest empirically with deep terminal S waves in Standard leads II and III and lead AVF, and a tall R wave in lead AVL (Diagram B of Fig. 103 and Fig. 71). Frontal plane axes in the region of 0° to −30° may at times be recorded from stocky or obese individuals, but may also reflect minor degrees of left anterior hemiblock. This requires substantiation.

Causes of left anterior hemiblock

Left anterior hemiblock may be due to the following causes:

(A) *Myocardial infarction*

Interruption of the anterosuperior division of the left bundle branch may be due to myocardial infarction. This results in *anterolateral peri-infarction block*. When this occurs, the initial vector is directed inferiorly and to the right, i.e. away from the infarcted anterolateral surface; an expression of the loss of forces due to the necrotic tissue itself. The terminal QRS forces are directed superiorly and to the left—the expression of the left anterior hemiblock (Diagram B of Fig. 110). See also section on Peri-infarction Block (page 106).

(B) *Fibrosis and calcareous encroachment*

Interruption of the anterosuperior division of the left bundle branch may be the result of fibrosis or calcareous encroachment from neighbouring structures (Diagram A in Fig. 110). This may be due to:

(i)   the fibrosis resulting from chronic coronary insufficiency.
(ii) the fibrosis resulting from chronic cardiac failure.
(iii) the fibrosis resulting from chronic left ventricular decompensation in cases of systemic hypertension and other diseases associated with left ventricular failure. *Note*: Left ventricular hypertrophy *per se* does not cause left axis deviation; it is rather the associated fibrosis which is responsible (Grant, 1957[3]).
(iv) fibrosis associated with a chronic cardiomyopathy.
(v)   calcareous encroachment on the left bundle branch conducting system from neighbouring structures such as the aortic valve and interventricular septum, also known as Lev's disease.[4]

Left posterior hemiblock

This results when conduction is interrupted in the postero-inferior division of the left bundle branch. When this occurs, the activation front of the postero-inferior division is lost, i.e. Vector 2 of Fig. 103 is abolished.

Activation now occurs predominantly through the fibres of the antero-superior division (Diagram C of Fig. 103). And since this activation

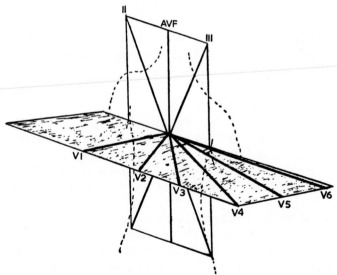

FIG. 104. Diagram illustrating the spatial orientation of the frontal and horizontal plane leads (see text).

front is directed downwards and to the right, the result is a *right axis deviation* (Fig. 26).

The mean manifest frontal plane QRS axis is rightwardly directed to the region of +90° to +120° on the hexaxial reference system (Vector 1 in Fig. 103). This results in prominent S waves in Standard lead I and lead AVL, and a tall R wave (of a qR complex) in Standard leads II, III and lead AVF. The R wave is particularly tall in Standard lead III. Other causes of right axis deviation, such as right ventricular dominance, must be excluded on both clinical and electrocardiographic grounds before the diagnosis of right posterior hemiblock can be established. Left posterior hemiblock is consequently not a pure electrocardiographic diagnosis, but always a clinical-electrocardiographic correlation. See also section on Peri-infarction Block (page 106).

FURTHER APPLICATION

SPECIFIC ORIENTATION OF THE LEAD AXES

FRONTAL AND HORIZONTAL PLANE LEADS

The twelve conventional electrocardiographic leads may be divided into two major groups on the basis of lead orientation (Fig. 104):

> Standard leads I, II and III, and leads AVR, AVL and AVF are orientated in the frontal plane and are termed the **frontal plane leads**.
>
> The precordial leads are orientated in the horizontal plane, i.e. at right angles to the frontal plane leads, and are termed the **horizontal plane leads**.

LEADS ORIENTATED TOWARDS THE CAVITY OF THE HEART

Lead AVR: The positive pole of lead AVR is usually orientated to the back of the atria and the cavities of the ventricles (Fig. 105). All impulses are therefore directed away from the positive pole of lead AVR; the P, QRS and T waves are therefore normally negative in this lead.

Lead V1: Lead V1 is orientated to the proximal region of the free wall of the right ventricle (Fig. 105). It therefore tends to be orientated towards the base, or even the cavity, of the heart. And, as with lead AVR, most deflections are, as a rule, predominantly negative in this lead. Thus, generally speaking, interpretation of abnormal electrocardiographic patterns is only based on positive deflections in this lead.

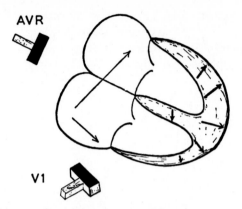

FIG. 105. Diagram illustrating the orientation of leads AVR and V1.

LEADS ORIENTATED TO THE ANTEROLATERAL SURFACE OF
THE HEART (Figs. 13, 27, 29 and 92)
Standard lead I.
Lead AVL.
Lateral precordial leads—leads V5 and V6.

Note: Lead V6—a horizontal plane lead—tends to be in the same plane as Standard lead I—a frontal plane lead (Fig. 104). Consequently, similar complexes are usually recorded by these leads.

LEADS ORIENTATED TO THE INFERIOR SURFACE OF THE
HEART (Figs. 13, 37, 93 and 94)
Standard leads II and III.
Lead AVF.

LEADS ORIENTATED TO THE ANTERIOR SURFACE OF THE
HEART (Figs. 13, 29 and 37)
Leads (V1) V2 to V6.

LEADS ORIENTATED TO THE RIGHT VENTRICLE (Fig. 33)
Leads V1, V2 (V3).

LEADS ORIENTATED TO THE LEFT VENTRICLE (Figs. 13 and 33)
Leads (V4) V5 and V6.
Standard lead I and lead AVL.

LEADS ORIENTATED TO THE ANTEROSEPTAL SURFACE OF THE
HEART (Figs. 13 and 29)
Usually leads V3 and V4.
These leads usually reflect the transition zone.

LEADS ORIENTATED TOWARDS THE DOMINANT VENTRICULAR MUSCLE MASS

In the frontal plane: Standard lead II (Fig. 106).

In the horizontal plane: Usually lead V5 (Fig. 107).

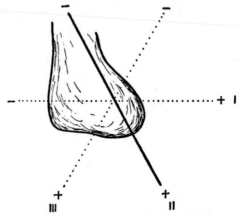

FIG. 106. Diagram illustrating the usual orientation of Standard lead II towards the main muscle mass of the ventricles.

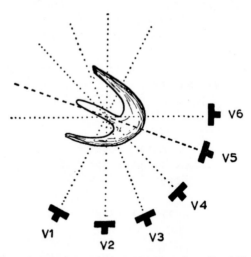

FIG. 107. Diagram illustrating the usual orientation of lead V5 towards the main muscle mass of the ventricles.

THE QRS-T ANGLE

The mean frontal plane QRS axis and the mean frontal plane T wave axis are usually similarly directed, i.e. they are close to each other; the angle between them is consequently narrow and does not normally exceed 60° (Fig. 108).

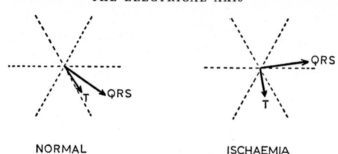

NORMAL   ISCHAEMIA

FIG. 108. Diagram illustrating the effect of myocardial ischaemia on the QRS-T angle. Normal: note the narrow QRS-T angle. Ischaemia: note the wide QRS-T angle.

In the presence of myocardial disease—commonly ischaemia—the T wave axis tends to deviate from the ischaemic region whereas the QRS axis usually remains normally directed, or may even deviate in the opposite direction (Fig. 108). The angle between the QRS and T wave axes therefore widens, and it is usually a sign of myocardial disease when it exceeds 60° in the adult.

Example I. The electrocardiogram shown in Fig. 101 has a normal QRS-T angle of 30° (QRS axis = +60°; T wave axis = +30°).

Example II. The electrocardiogram shown in Fig. 51 has a wide and abnormal QRS-T angle of 70° (QRS axis = 0°; T wave axis = +70°).

Note: This causes the T wave to be taller in Standard lead III than in Standard lead I.

The QRS-T angle is thus a sensitive index of significant T wave abnormality and is more reliable than the empirical observation of T wave change in isolated leads.

Digitalis effect and the QRS-T angle
Digitalis effect will diminish the magnitude of the T wave axis but will not change its direction. Thus, an abnormally wide QRS-T angle in a patient receiving digitalis indicates that the abnormality was present before the administration of the digitalis.

The horizontal plane QRS-T angle
A wide QRS-T angle may also be reflected in the horizontal plane leads. The main horizontal plane QRS and T wave forces are normally directed towards lead V6 and away from lead V1 (Fig. 109). The QRS complex and T wave are therefore normally upright in lead V6 and negative in lead V1. Coronary insufficiency causes the T wave forces to deviate away from the QRS forces (Fig. 109). In the early stages of this deviation (dotted arrows in Fig. 109), the T wave force may be more

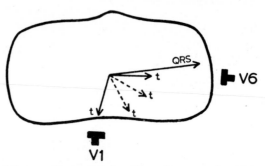

FIG. 109. Diagram illustrating the effects of coronary insufficiency on the horizontal plane QRS-T angle (see text).

orientated towards lead V1 than lead V6 and the *T wave in lead V1 thus becomes taller than the T wave in lead V6*; the QRS complex remains directed to lead V6 which still records a tall R wave. This wide angle between the QRS and T wave forces in the horizontal plane—resulting in a *T-V1 taller than T-V6 syndrome*—may be the earliest sign of coronary insufficiency (see also page 44). Caution must, however, be exercised in the interpretation of the *T-V1 taller than T-V6 syndrowe*, since errors in electrode placement can effect the same result. The QRS-T angle eventually becomes wider still and the T wave becomes frankly inverted in lead V6 and dominantly upright in lead V1.

THE INITIAL AND TERMINAL QRS FORCES

The mean QRS axis refers to the dominant, average or general direction of the QRS forces. Under certain circumstances, however, it is of value to consider the direction of the initial and terminal QRS forces separately. The direction of the first part of the QRS deflection is determined by only taking note of the first 0.04 sec of the QRS deflection in all the frontal plane leads, and ascertaining the direction of this initial vector in a manner similar to that used for the mean QRS axis (Grant, 1957[3]). The vector for the terminal 0.04 sec of the QRS deflection is similarly determined.

These initial and terminal forces may be compared with each other, as well as with the mean QRS axis. This may reveal such conditions as *peri-infarction block* and the S1, S2, S3 syndrome.

PERI-INFARCTION BLOCK AND THE VECTOR PRINCIPLES OF MYOCARDIAL INFARCTION

THE INITIAL 0.04 VECTOR

As indicated previously, the QRS forces are *directed away from the necrotic area of myocardial infarction* (see page 18 and Fig. 21). It is particularly the initial QRS forces that are directed away from the infarcted area, and leads orientated to this area will consequently record deep, wide pathological Q waves. Thus, a deep, wide Q wave is, in effect, a reflection of the initial 0.04 QRS vector being directed away from the positive pole of the lead. In inferior myocardial infarction, the initial QRS force moves away from the inferior or diaphragmatic surface of the heart, and leads orientated to this surface (Standard leads II, III and lead AVF) will reflect deep, wide Q waves. Viewed vectorially, the initial vector will be located in the region of $-60°$ to $-100°$ on the hexaxial reference system (vector i in Diagram C of Fig. 110).

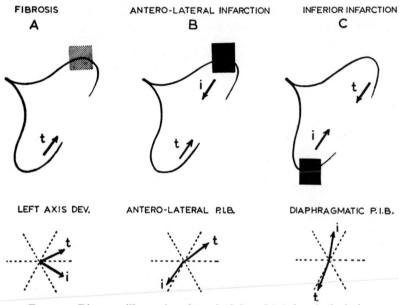

FIG. 110. Diagram illustrating the principles of A left axis deviation, B anterolateral peri-infarction block, C diaphragmatic peri-infarction block (see text).

Example I. With reference to Fig. 111.

When only the initial 0.04 part of the QRS deflection is considered, the largest deflection occurs in Standard lead III and is negative in this lead (Fig. 111); the initial 0.04 part of the QRS complex is almost equiphasic in lead AVR. See also Fig. 112. The initial vector is thus located at $-60°$, i.e. away from the inferior wall of the ventricles.

Example II. With reference to Fig. 113.

When only the initial 0.04 part of the QRS deflection is considered, the largest deflection occurs in lead AVF and is positive in this lead;

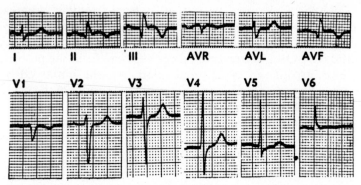

FIG. 111. Electrocardiogram illustrating acute inferolateral myocardial infarction with diaphragmatic peri-infarction block. Note pathological Q waves, raised convex-upward S-T segments and inverted T waves in Standard leads II, III and lead AVF, and raised S-T segment and inverted T wave in lead V6, indicating inferolateral infarction. Initial QRS vector is located at −60°; the terminal QRS vector is located at +120° (see text and Fig. 112).

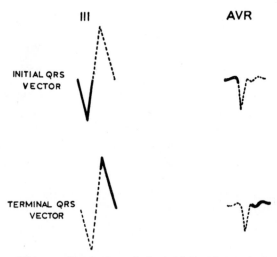

FIG. 112. Diagram illustration of the initial and terminal 0.04 sec QRS vectors as reflected in Standard leads III and AVR of Fig. 111.

the initial 0.04 part of the QRS complex is equiphasic in Standard lead I. The initial vector is thus located at +90°.

THE TERMINAL 0.04 VECTOR

As indicated previously, the left bundle branch divides into two major sweeps or radiations: the anterosuperior division and the postero-

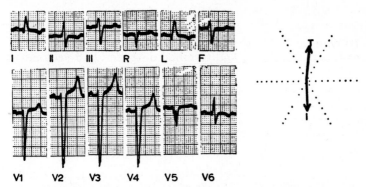

FIG. 113. Electrocardiogram illustrating the features of anterolateral peri-infarction block. Initial vector (labelled I) located at +90° on the hexaxial reference system. Terminal vector (labelled T) located at −80° on the hexaxial reference system (see text).

inferior division (Figs. 102, 103, 110). If conduction is interrupted in the branches of the anterosuperior division (Fig. 103 and Diagrams A and B of Fig. 110) activation of the ventricles will be effected principally through the branches of the postero-inferior division; the vector will therefore be directed upwards and to the left. This deviation affects principally the terminal 0.04 vector, i.e. there is a terminal left axis deviation. This type of interruption may be due to *fibrosis* or *infarction* involving the anterolateral aspect of the left ventricle. It will be noted that in the case of infarction, the *terminal vector points towards the infarcted area.*

If conduction is interrupted in the branches of the postero-inferior division of the left bundle branch, activation of the ventricles will be effected principally through the branches of the anterosuperior division; the terminal vector will then be directed downwards and to the right (vector t in Diagram C of Fig. 110), i.e. there is a terminal right axis deviation.

Interruption of the postero-inferior division is mainly due to inferior myocardial infarction, and it is noteworthy that the *terminal vector is again directed towards the infarcted area.*

Example I. With reference to Fig. 111.

The largest deflection of the terminal 0.04 sec of the QRS complex occurs in Standard lead III and is positive in this lead; the most equiphasic deflection of the terminal 0.04 sec of the QRS complex occurs in lead AVR. The terminal 0.04 sec vector is therefore located at +120°. These principles are diagrammatically illustrated in Diagram C of Fig. 110 and Fig. 112.

Summary of QRS vectors in Fig. 111
>   Initial 0.04 sec QRS vector located at −60°.
>   Terminal 0.04 sec QRS vector located at +120°.
>   Angle between initial and terminal 0.04 sec QRS vectors: 180°.

Example II. With reference to Fig. 113.
The largest deflection of the terminal 0.04 sec of the QRS complex occurs in lead AVF and is negative in this lead; the most equiphasic deflection occurs in Standard lead I (it is slightly more positive than negative). The terminal vector is therefore located at −80°.

Summary of QRS vectors in Fig. 113
>   Initial 0.04 sec QRS vector located at +90°.
>   Terminal 0.04 sec QRS vector located at −80°.
>   Angle between initial terminal 0.04 sec QRS vectors: 170°.

On the basis of the aforementioned principles, it will be noted that (a) the initial 0.04 QRS vector is directed *away* from the infarcted area, and (b) when the infarct interrupts either the anterosuperior or postero-inferior divisions of the left bundle branch, the terminal 0.04 sec QRS vector is directed *towards* the infarcted area. This will result in a *wide angle—greater than* 100°—*between the initial and terminal QRS vectors* and is termed **peri-infarction block**.

When an anterolateral infarction interrupts the anterosuperior division of the left bundle branch, the initial vector is directed downwards and to the right, and the terminal vector is directed upwards and to the left (Diagram B of Fig. 110). This is termed **anterolateral peri-infarction block**.

When an inferior infarction interrupts the postero-inferior division of the left bundle branch, the initial vector is directed upwards and to the left, and the terminal vector is directed downwards and to the right (Diagram C of Fig. 110). This is termed **diaphragmatic peri-infarction block**.

Note: When left axis deviation is due to fibrosis only, the angle between the initial and terminal QRS forces is narrow.

SUMMARY OF THE VECTOR PRINCIPLES IN
MYOCARDIAL INFARCTION
(Fig. 114)

1. The initial QRS vector is directed away from the infarcted area (vector 1 in Fig. 114). This results in a deep, wide pathological Q wave in leads directed towards the infarcted area.
2. The terminal QRS vector is directed towards the infarcted area

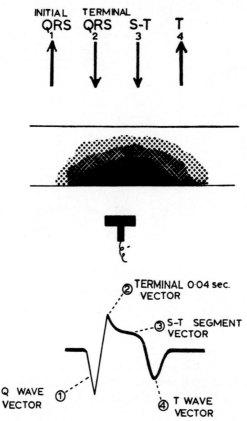

FIG. 114. Diagram illustrating the vector principles of myocardial infarction (see text).

(vector 2 in Fig. 114). This only occurs in some cases of antero-lateral and inferior myocardial infarctions.

3. The S-T segment vector is directed towards the infarcted area (vector 3 in Fig. 114). This results in a raised S-T segment in leads orientated towards the infarcted area.

4. The T wave vector is directed away from the infarcted area (vector 4 in Fig. 114). This results in an inverted T wave in leads orientated towards the infarcted area.

THE VECTORAL SIGNIFICANCE OF A Q WAVE IN STANDARD LEAD III

A Q wave in Standard lead III is often a sign of old inferior myocardial infarction. However, a Q wave in this lead may also occur normally. Vectorial evaluation will assist in the differentiation.

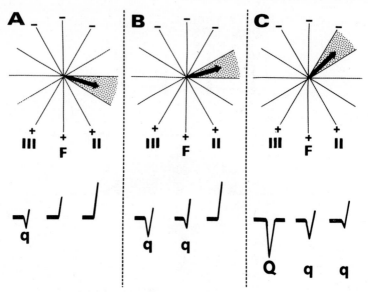

FIG. 115. Diagrams illustrating the vectorial significance of a Q wave in Standard lead III.

A Q wave will appear in Standard lead III if the initial vector is situated anywhere in the hemisphere between +30° counter-clockwise to −150° on the hexaxial reference system. When this occurs, the initial vector will always be orientated towards the negative pole of the Standard lead III lead axis.

When the initial QRS vector is situated in the region of 0° to +30°, a Q wave will appear in Standard lead III *only*, i.e. there will be no Q waves in lead AVF or Standard lead II as the vector is directed towards the positive poles of these leads (Diagram A of Fig. 115). This vector is directed laterally and to the left, i.e. it is not directed away from the inferior wall of the ventricle and is therefore not likely to be significant of myocardial infarction. In other words, a Q wave which appears in Standard lead III only is unlikely to be an expression of myocardial infarction.

When the initial QRS vector is situated in the region 0° to −30° (Diagram B of Fig. 115) it is directed towards the negative poles of Standard lead III *and* lead AVF, and a Q wave will be recorded by both these leads. This initial vector is directed laterally and to the left, i.e. it is *not* directed away from the inferior wall of the ventricle, and is therefore not likely to be significant of inferior myocardial infarction.

When the initial QRS vector is situated in the region of −30° counter-clockwise to −150° (Diagram C of Fig. 115) it is directed towards the negative poles of Standard leads II, III and lead AVF, and a Q wave will appear in all these leads. Furthermore, the initial QRS vector is now directed superiorly, i.e. away from the inferior wall of the ventricle and may thus be indicative of inferior myocardial infarction.

Thus, a Q wave in Standard lead III is significant of inferior myocardial infarction under the following circumstances:

(a) When it is *associated with a Q wave in Standard lead II and lead AVF.*
(b) When it fulfils the criteria of size and duration for a pathological Q wave (page 35).

Note: Marked left axis deviation of the mean QRS axis, e.g. $-70°$, will result in dominantly negative deflections in Standard leads II and III, and lead AVF, which may, at times, mimic pathological Q waves.

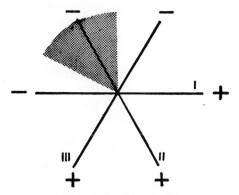

FIG. 116. The hexaxial reference system. The shaded area denotes the region of negativity for all three Standard leads, i.e. the location of the terminal QRS vector in the S1, S2, S3 syndrome.

THE S1, S2, S3 SYNDROME

This syndrome is characterized by a terminal vector that is directed *superiorly and to the right*, i.e. a vector located in the region of $-90°$ counter-clockwise to $-150°$ on the hexaxial system (Fig. 116). This vector is in the area of negativity for all the Standard leads and will thus produce prominent S waves in all the Standard leads (Fig. 117). The mean QRS axis is usually normal in direction.

This syndrome may be found in the following conditions (Grant, 1957[3]):

1. It may be a **normal** characteristic, and probably represents persistence of the juvenile pattern of right ventricular dominance (see below).
2. It may be associated with **right ventricular hypertrophy** and is believed to represent hypertrophy of the right ventricular outflow

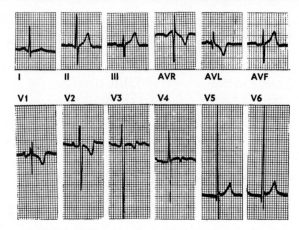

FIG. 117. Electrocardiogram illustrating the S1, S2, S3 syndrome.

tract—the *crista supraventricularis*. *Note*: the S1, S2, S3 syndrome constitutes supportive but not diagnostic evidence of right ventricular hypertrophy.

3. It may occasionally be associated with **myocardial infarction**; there will, however, always be other evidence of myocardial infarction, i.e. deformity of the initial QRS vector and/or S-T segment and T wave changes.

THE P WAVE AXIS

THE NORMAL P WAVE AXIS

The normal P wave axis is usually directed in the region of $+30°$ to $+60°$ on the frontal plane hexaxial reference system (Diagram A of Fig. 118).

THE ABNORMAL P WAVE AXIS

A. *P. pulmonale and P. congenitale*

Right atrial enlargement is associated with a tall peaked P wave in Standard lead II (page 85). This form of P wave may be found in association with either acquired or congenital heart disease. The P wave associated with each condition may be differentiated on a vectorial basis as follows (Sodi-Pallares & Calder, 1956[8]):

P. pulmonale. When P wave enlargement is associated with acquired heart disease, the P wave vector is usually directed in the region of $+60°$ to $+90°$ on the hexaxial reference system (Diagram B of Fig. 118). When the acquired heart disease is emphysema, the P wave axis is

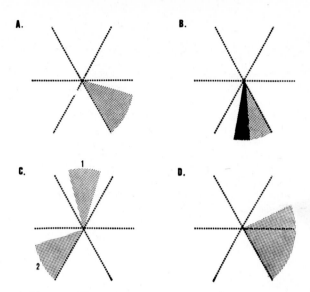

Fig. 118. Diagrams illustrating the distribution of P wave axes in various conditions. A. Normal range. B. Acquired right heart disease—*P. pulmonale.* Black shading represents the range for emphysema. C1. Retrograde atrial activation. C2. 'Mirror-image' dextrocardia or reversed arm electrodes. D. Congenital heart disease—*P. congenitale.*

usually in the region of $+90°$ (black shading in Diagram B of Fig. 118). **P. congenitale.** When P wave enlargement is associated with congenital heart disease, the P wave vector is usually directed in the region of $-30°$ to $+60°$ on the hexaxial reference system, i.e. the P wave axis rarely deviates further to the right than $+60°$ (Diagram D of Fig. 118).

B. *The P wave axis of retrograde atrial activation*
Retrograde atrial activation may occur with impulses of A-V nodal or ventricular origin. Retrograde atrial activation may also be associated with reciprocal rhythm of atrial origin where the sinus impulse, during its passage through the A-V node enters an A-V nodal by-pass and returns retrogradely to activate the atria a second time. Retrograde activation of the atria is directed cranially, and is thus associated with a superiorly directed P′ wave axis, i.e. an axis in the region of $-80°$ to $-100°$ (Diagram C1 of Fig. 118).

C. *'Mirror-image' dextrocardia*
In 'mirror-image' dextrocardia, the P wave axis is directed to the right, in the region of $+120°$ to $+150°$ (Diagram C2 of Fig. 118). A similar P wave axis will occur when the right and left arm electrodes are reversed.

REFERENCES

1 DAVIES J. N. P. & EVANS W. (1960) The significance of deep S waves in leads II and III. *Brit. Heart J.* **22,** 55.
2 GRANT R. P. (1956) Left axis deviation. *Circulation* **14,** 233.
3 GRANT R. P. (1957) *Clinical Electrocardiography.* New York: McGraw-Hill.
4 LEV M. (1964) Anatomic basis for atrioventricular block. *Amer. J. Med.* **37,** 742.
5 ROSENBAUM M. B. (1968) Types of right bundle branch block and their clinical significance. *J. Electrocardiol.* **1,** 221.
6 ROSENBAUM M. B. (1970) In *Symposium on Cardiac Arrhythmias,* ed. Sandoe E., Flensted-Jensen E. & Olesen K. H. Sodertalje, Sweden: A.B. Astra.
7 ROSENBAUM M. B., ELIZARI M. V. & LAZZARI J. O. (1970) *The Hemiblocks.* Oldsmar, Florida: Tampa Tracings.
8 SODI-PALLARES D. & CALDER R. M. (1956) *New Bases of Electrocardiography.* St. Louis, Illinois: C.V. Mosby Company.

CHAPTER 8

Hypothermia

Hypothermia manifests electrocardiographically as follows (illustrated in Fig. 119):

1. *Sinus bradycardia.* The result of a profound depression of pacemaker automaticity.
2. *Muscle tremor—'shivering'—artifact.*
3. *J wave.* This is a rounded, rather narrow, 'hump-like' wave usually superimposed on the distal limb of the QRS complex, and thought to be due to early repolarization.
4. *Prolonged Q–T interval.*

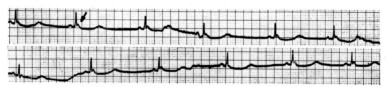

FIG. 119. Electrocardiogram (continuous strip of Standard lead II) showing the features of hypothermia. *Note*: 1. Sinus bradycardia. 2. The *J* wave (example illustrated with arrow). 3. 'Shivering'—muscle tremor—artifact. 4. Prolonged Q–T interval.

PART II

Disorders of Cardiac Rhythm

Basic Principles

CHAPTER 9

Basic Principles

The electrocardiogram is conventionally recorded at a speed of 25 mm per second. The electrocardiographic paper is divided into large and small squares (Fig. 120).

Each large square represents 0.20 sec
Five large squares represent 1 sec
Fifteen large squares represent 3 sec
Each small square represents 0.04 ($\frac{1}{25}$) sec

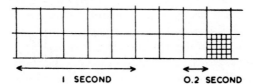

I SECOND   0.2 SECOND

FIG. 120. Electrocardiographic graph paper.

The cardiac rate may be estimated by counting the number of cardiac cycles—R–R intervals—in fifteen squares (3 sec) and multiplying by 20.

Note: Most recording graphs have every fifteenth large square marked by a vertical line at the border of the recording paper (Fig. 122).

ANATOMY AND PHYSIOLOGY OF THE CONDUCTING SYSTEM

The rate and rhythm of the heart are controlled by the **sino-atrial node (S-A node)**, which is situated in the wall of the right atrium to the right of the superior vena caval orifice (Fig. 2). The sinus impulse leaves the S-A node and spreads through the atrial muscle; this atrial activation is reflected by the P wave of the electrocardiogram. The sinus impulse eventually reaches the A-V node which is situated in the right atrium above the tricuspid valve and just to the right of the interatrial septum. After a delay at the A-V node (reflected in the electrocardiogram as the greater part of the P–R interval) the impulse travels down the bundle of His, bundle branches and Purkinje network system. The **bundle of His** passes horizontally to the left from the A-V node, pierces the membranous interventricular septum and divides into **right and left bundle branches**. These pass down on either side of the muscular interventricular septum and finally divide into the **Purkinje network of fibres** which proceed vertically to the surface of the heart from the endocardium to the epicardium (see also page 5 and Figs. 2 and 4).

The S-A node is under the influence of the vagus nerve and normal variations in heart rate are effected mainly by variations in vagal tone. An *increase* in vagal tone slows the heart; a *decrease* in vagal tone accelerates the heart.

THE PACEMAKERS OF THE HEART

The heart has many potential pacemaking cells. These are situated in the S-A node, the A-V node, the bundle of His, and the ventricles (every Purkinje cell is a potential pacemaking cell). The S-A node has the fastest inherent discharge rate which usually ranges from 70 to 80 beats per minute. The inherent rate of potential A-V nodal pacemaking cells is about 60 beats per minute. The inherent rate of pacemaking cells in the bundle of His is about 50 beats per minute. The inherent rate of the Purkinje cells of the ventricular muscle is about 30 to 40 beats per minute. In other words, the more distal a potential pacemaker is situated from the S-A node, the slower its inherent discharge rate.

There is, however, only one pacemaker that is normally in control of the heart. This is the S-A node, the pacemaker with the fastest inherent discharge rate. Its impulse reaches the slower subsidiary pacemakers before they have an opportunity to mature and 'fire' spontaneously, and discharges them prematurely. Thus, the slower potential pacemaking cells enjoy *no protection* from the impulses of the fastest pacemaker.

CLASSIFICATION OF THE ARRHYTHMIAS

1. DISTURBANCES OF IMPULSE FORMATION

Sinus rhythms
    Sinus arrhythmia
    Sinus tachycardia
    Sinus bradycardia

Ectopic atrial rhythms
>   Atrial extrasystoles
>   Paroxysmal atrial tachycardia
>   Atrial fibrillation
>   Atrial flutter
>   Atrial escape

A-V nodal rhythms
>   A-V nodal extrasystoles
>   Extrasystolic—paroxysmal—A-V nodal tachycardia
>   Idionodal tachycardia
>   A-V nodal escape

Ventricular rhythms
>   Ventricular extrasystoles
>   Extrasystolic ventricular tachycardia
>   Idioventricular tachycardia
>   Ventricular flutter
>   Ventricular fibrillation
>   Ventricular parasystole
>   Ventricular escape

2. DISTURBANCES OF IMPULSE CONDUCTION

S-A block
A-V block
Phasic aberrant ventricular conduction

Disorders of Impulse Formation

CHAPTER 10

Sinus Rhythms

SINUS ARRHYTHMIA · SINUS TACHYCARDIA ·
SINUS BRADYCARDIA

SINUS ARRHYTHMIA

Sinus arrhythmia is characterized by alternating periods of slow and rapid rates; it is due to an irregular discharge of the S-A node. The condition is most commonly associated with the phases of respiration— **respiratory sinus arrhythmia**. The periods of faster rate occur towards the end of inspiration, and the periods of slower rate towards the end of expiration. The mechanism is mediated by reflex stimulation of the vagus nerve from receptors in the lungs.

Diagnosis. The impulses arise from the S-A node and the P waves are therefore normal; the subsequent course of the sinus impulse is also normal, resulting in a normal P–R interval and QRST complex. The arrhythmia is thus characterized by **normal P-QRST complexes** with alternating periods of gradually lengthening and gradually shortening P–P intervals (Fig. 121).

Sinus arrhythmia is accentuated by vagotonic procedures, viz. digitalis administration, carotid sinus and eyeball compression. It is abolished by vagolytic procedures, viz. exercise, atropine and amyl nitrite.

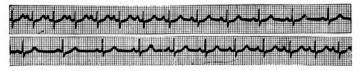

FIG. 121. Electrocardiogram (continuous recording—Standard lead II) showing sinus arrhythmia.

Respiratory sinus arrhythmia is a normal physiological phenomenon, and is most marked in young persons.

SINUS TACHYCARDIA

Sinus tachycardia occurs when the S-A node discharges at a rate faster than 100 per minute in the adult. (In infants the normal 'resting' rate averages 120–130 beats per minute, slowing gradually to reach the adult rate at puberty.)

Diagnosis. Sinus tachycardia is characterized by **normal P-QRST complexes which are recorded in rapid succession**. It varies with emotion, respiration and exercise. Vagotonic procedures, e.g. eyeball and carotid sinus compression, result in slight but gradual slowing.

SIGNIFICANCE
Sinus tachycardia is the normal physiological response to exercise and emotion. It is the reaction to cardiac failure, fever, thyrotoxicosis and anaemia. It may be caused by the administration of adrenaline, atropine, caffeine and amyl nitrate.

SINUS BRADYCARDIA

Sinus bradycardia occurs when the S-A node discharges at a rate slower than 60 per minute.

Diagnosis. Sinus bradycardia is characterized by **normal P-QRST complexes which are recorded in slow succession** (Fig. 122). It is commonly associated with respiratory sinus arrhythmia.

SIGNIFICANCE
Sinus bradycardia occurs as a normal variation in athletes. Slowing of the sinus rate—at times to bradycardic levels—is the physiological

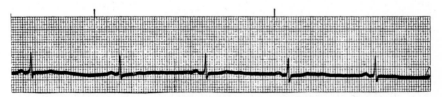

FIG. 122. Electrocardiogram showing marked sinus bradycardia. *Note:* there are just over two cardiac cycles, or R–R intervals, in every 3 sec— fifteen large squares (every fifteenth large square is marked by a vertical line on the upper border of the graph paper); the rate is therefore just over 40 per minute.

response to sleep. Sinus bradycardia is accentuated by digitalis and vagotonic procedures (eyeball and carotid sinus compression); the rate quickens gradually with exercise, emotion and amyl nitrite.

Sinus bradycardia is associated with myxoedema, obstructive jaundice (the effect of direct action of the bile salts on the S-A node), increased intracranial pressure and glaucoma (increased and persistent oculocardiac reflex).

See also the differential diagnosis of a slow regular ventricular rhythm (page 220).

CHAPTER II

Ectopic Atrial Rhythms

ATRIAL EXTRASYSTOLES · PAROXYSMAL ATRIAL TACHY-
CARDIA · ATRIAL FIBRILLATION · ATRIAL FLUTTER ·
ATRIAL ESCAPE

ATRIAL EXTRASYSTOLES

An atrial extrasystole is due to the **premature** discharge of an **ectopic atrial focus**. It has the following characteristics:

1. THE P WAVE IS BIZARRE

The discharge arises from an ectopic atrial focus, i.e. from a point other than the S-A node. It thus travels across the atria by unusual pathways resulting in an abnormal or bizarre P′ wave—a P′ wave that is different from the sinus P wave and which may be *pointed, diphasic* or *inverted* (Figs. 123, 124B, 125 and 159).

2. THE BIZARRE P′ WAVE IS PREMATURE

The ectopic impulses arise in the diastolic period of the preceding sinus beat and is thus recorded earlier than the next anticipated sinus P wave.

3. THE COMPENSATORY PAUSE IS INCOMPLETE (see Fig. 123)

(*a*) The ectopic impulse reaches and discharges the sinus node prematurely—position A in Fig. 123.

(*b*) The recharge of the S-A node thus begins at position A and the next sinus discharge occurs at position C. (Had the sinus node not been prematurely discharged, the recharge would begin at position B and the following discharge would then occur at position D.)

(*c*) The next normal sinus impulse therefore does not occur as scheduled, viz. at position B; for the S-A node must pass through a *complete recovery cycle* before it can discharge again.

(*d*) The basic rhythm of the S-A node is thus disturbed and a pause follows the ectopic beat—the compensatory pause. This pause, however, is incomplete, i.e. it does not fully compensate for the prematurity of the extrasystole. This means that the sum of the pre- and post-ectopic intervals (Y–Z in Figs. 123 and 124) is *less than* the sum of two consecutive normal intervals (X–Y in Figs. 123 and 124).

Compare these events with those occasioned by a ventricular

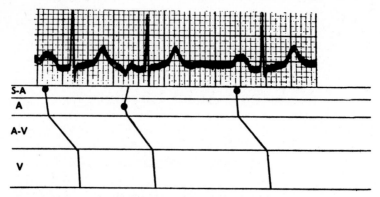

FIG. 123. Electrocardiogram (Standard lead II) showing (*a*) an atrial extrasystole—note the bizarre premature P wave; (*b*) first degree A-V block of the sinus impulse: P–R interval = 0.24 sec (six small squares); (*c*) **P. mitrale**—the sinus P wave is widened and plateau-shaped. From a case of mitral stenosis on digitalis therapy. The large black dots indicate impulse origin. S-A = sino-atrial level; A = atrial level; A-V = A-V nodal level; V = ventricular level.

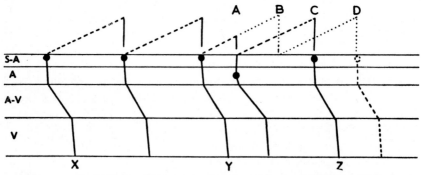

FIG. 124A. Diagram illustrating the disturbance of rhythm which occurs with an atrial extrasystole. The dotted lines indicate the recharge of the S-A node. The large black dots indicate impulse origin (see text).

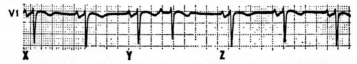

FIG. 124B. Electrocardiogram (lead V1) showing normal sinus rhythm complicated by an atrial extrasystole. This is reflected by the fourth P wave which is premature and bizarre. The compensatory pause is incomplete, i.e. the sum of the pre- and post-ectopic intervals (interval Y–Z) is *less than* the sum of two consecutive sinus intervals (interval X–Y).

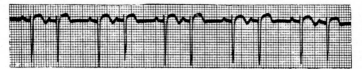

Fig. 125. Electrocardiogram showing alternate atrial extrasystoles causing bigeminal rhythm.

extrasystole where the sinus rhythm is not disturbed and where the compensatory pause is consequently complete (Fig. 140).

4. CONDUCTION OF THE ECTOPIC ATRIAL IMPULSE

(a) A-V conduction

Conduction of the atrial impulse to the ventricles depends upon the recovery state of the A-V node when the impulse reaches it. Thus:

(i) The ectopic impulse may be *blocked*: A very early impulse may find the A-V node refractory and conduction to the ventricles is therefore blocked. A blocked or non-conducted atrial extrasystole is characterized by an abnormal and premature P wave that is *not* followed by a QRS complex (Figs. 57, 155 and 173). The abnormal P wave may not be obvious, especially if it is superimposed on the T wave of the preceding sinus beat; as a result, the T wave is slightly deformed—a little more pointed or slightly notched (Fig. 173, top strip). And if this premature abnormal P wave is not observed, the pause may be mistakenly diagnosed as due to S-A block. Thus, in all cases where a long pause is apparently due to S-A block, the preceding T wave must be compared with other T waves and critically examined for even the slightest deformity.

(ii) The atrial impulse may be conducted with:

   (a) A *normal P–R interval* (Fig. 125).
   (b) A *prolonged P–R interval*; this will occur if the extrasystole is early and thus finds the A-V node only partially recovered.
   (c) A *relatively short P–R interval*, i.e. a P–R interval that is shorter than that of the conducted sinus beat (Fig. 123); this will occur when the extrasystole arises from a focus that is relatively low in the atria and thus reaches the A-V node quickly.

(b) Intraventricular conduction

After passing through the A-V node the ectopic impulse may be conducted to the ventricles as follows:

(i) With *normal intraventricular conduction*: the impulse is conducted through both bundle branches and results in a normal QRS complex (Figs. 123, 125 and 126).

(ii) With *aberrant ventricular conduction*: the impulse reaches the bundle branches when only one has fully recovered. The impulse is then conducted through one bundle branch only resulting in a bizarre QRS complex (Figs. 173 and 175, and see Chapter 18 on Phasic Aberrant Ventricular Conduction).

SIGNIFICANCE OF ATRIAL EXTRASYSTOLES

Atrial extrasystoles may be found in association with *chronic rheumatic valvular disease*—mitral stenosis and mitral incompetence; in coronary artery disease, in thyrotoxicosis and in digitalis intoxication. Frequent multifocal atrial extrasystoles often herald atrial fibrillation. Three or more consecutive atrial extrasystoles constitute a paroxysmal atrial tachycardia. Occasional atrial extrasystoles may occur in normal individuals.

Alternate atrial extrasystoles are a cause of bigeminal rhythm (Fig. 125).

SUMMARY

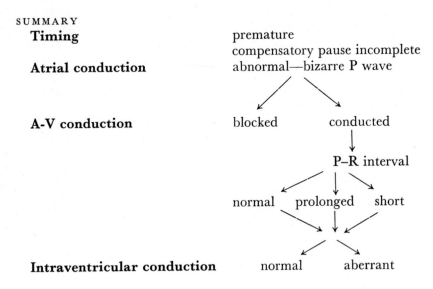

Timing   premature
                              compensatory pause incomplete
Atrial conduction   abnormal—bizarre P wave

A-V conduction   blocked   conducted

                                                     P–R interval

                              normal   prolonged   short

Intraventricular conduction   normal   aberrant

EXTRASYSTOLIC—PAROXYSMAL—ATRIAL TACHYCARDIA

Paroxysmal atrial tachycardia is due to the rapid discharge of an ectopic atrial focus: a series of three or more rapidly occurring, regular and consecutive atrial extrasystoles.

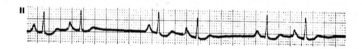

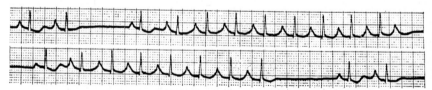

FIG. 126. *Top strip*: Electrocardiogram (Standard lead II) showing sinus rhythm complicated by alternate atrial extrasystoles resulting in bigeminal rhythm.

Bottom two strips: (continuous recording; a later section of the same electrocardiogram) showing sinus rhythm with atrial extrasystoles (beginning and end of the record), and two paroxysms of extrasystolic atrial tachycardia arising from the same ectopic atrial focus as the atrial extrasystoles.

MECHANISM AND ELECTROCARDIOGRAPHIC CHARACTERISTICS

1. Atrial activation.

   The atrial focus is ectopic and the course of atrial depolarization is therefore abnormal. This results in an *abnormally shaped* P wave (Fig. 126).

2. A-V conduction.

   On reaching the A-V node, the atrial impulse may be conducted as follows:

   (*a*) With *normal A-V conduction*—normal P–R interval.

   (*b*) With *first degree A-V block*.

   Because of the rapid ectopic discharge rate and conduction frequency through the A-V node there is insufficient time for complete recovery of the A-V node. The atrial impulse is thus conducted with first degree A-V block (Fig. 126).

   (*c*) With *second degree A-V block*.

   The ectopic discharge may be so rapid that every second atrial impulse is blocked—a 2:1 A-V block.

   At times the atrial tachycardia is associated with more complex forms of second degree A-V block, e.g. (*a*) a 3:2 block, possibly of the Wenckebach type or (*b*) a fluctuating ratio in the degree of A-V block, e.g. 3:2, 2:1, 2:1, 3:2, etc. (Fig. 127). This form is frequently due to digitalis intoxication, and is sometimes abbreviated to the cryptic term of 'P.A.T. with block'.

3. (a) With *normal intraventricular conduction*.

Intraventricular conduction may be normal. This will manifest with a series of normal QRS complexes which are inscribed in rapid and regular succession, each related to an ectopic atrial P wave (Figs. 126 and 127).

(b) With *phasic aberrant ventricular conduction*

The impulses of the atrial tachycardia may be conducted with phasic aberrant ventricular conduction (see Chapter 18). The atrial impulses are conducted through one bundle branch only resulting in the bizarre QRS complex of right or left bundle branch block (see Chapter 18). This may mimic paroxysmal ventricular tachycardia (Figs. 177 and 180).

4. The effect on the S-T segment and T wave.

Any tachycardia may result in relative coronary insufficiency, which will of course be worse if the coronary arteries are diseased. The coronary insufficiency manifests as S-T segment depression and T wave inversion. These changes are present during the tachycardia and may persist for hours or days *after the tachycardia has ceased*—the **post-tachycardia syndrome**.

SUPRAVENTRICULAR TACHYCARDIA

When identification of the P′ waves is difficult, or the P′ to QRS relationship cannot be established with certainty the rhythm may be conveniently referred to as **paroxysmal supraventricular tachycardia**.

SUMMARY

Atrial conduction: Abnormal P waves *preceding* the QRS complexes (recognition of P waves often difficult)

A-V conduction: first degree   second degree   normal
                     A-V block   A-V block   conduction
                                              (uncommon)

Intraventricular conduction: normal   ←   aberrant

S-T segment: frequently depressed

T wave: frequently inverted

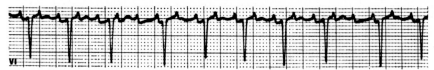

FIG. 127. Electrocardiogram (lead V1) showing extrasystolic atrial tachycardia with varying second degree A-V block: 'P.A.T. with block'.

ATRIAL FIBRILLATION

Under normal circumstances the sinus impulse is transmitted uniformly, evenly and concentrically to all parts of the atria. In atrial fibrillation *excitation and recovery of the atria are disorganized and chaotic*. The atria are functionally fractionated into a chaotic state of numerous tissue islets in various stages of excitation and recovery. These numerous excitatory wavelets or stimuli course irregularly through atria and reach the A-V node at frequent and irregular intervals. The A-V node can only conduct some of these stimuli, because, following conduction of one such stimulus, it is refractory for a short period, and impulses reaching the A-V node during this period are blocked. As the refractory period of the A-V node varies with such factors as vagal stimulation, respiration, emotion, exercise, and incomplete or partial penetration of the atrial impulses into the A-V node (concealed conduction), transmission to the ventricles is irregular.

The impulses from the fibrillating atria may, at times, be conducted to the ventricles with phasic aberrant ventricular conduction (see Chapter 18).

In untreated cases the ventricular response, i.e. the ventricular rate is usually about 120–150 per minute. Digitalis slows, i.e. diminishes the ventricular response by *increasing the refractory period of the A-V node*.

The initiation of atrial fibrillation is the result of *very early stimulation* of the atria, and is usually due to a very premature atrial extrasystole (Fig. 129). Maintenance of the fibrillation is favoured by a *large mass of atrial tissue*.

ELECTROCARDIOGRAPHIC MANIFESTATIONS

The atrial deflections are irregular and chaotic resulting in a *ragged baseline* with numerous rounded or spiked waves of varying shape, height and width (Fig. 128).

In long-standing cases of atrial fibrillation the deflections may be of low amplitude and the baseline may be almost straight with minimal smooth low-amplitude undulations (Fig. 128A).

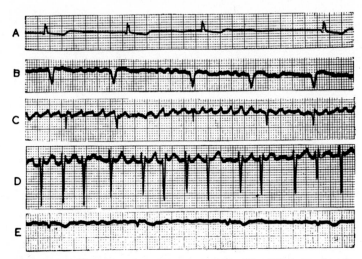

FIG. 128. Electrocardiograms (all tracings are of lead Vi) showing the various manifestations of atrial fibrillation (A) shows long-standing atrial fibrillation. Note (*a*) the smooth, slightly undulating baseline; (*b*) the slow and irregular ventricular response; (*c*) the digitalis effect in the S-T segment. (B) and (C) are examples of a coarser, more recent fibrillation with a relatively slow ventricular response. Note the irregular and ragged baseline. (D) shows the same features as (C) but with a rapid ventricular response. (E) shows atrial fibrillation with complete A-V block. Note the *regularly* spaced QRS complexes.

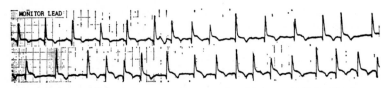

FIG. 129. Electrocardiogram (Monitor lead) showing: 1. Sinus rhythm. This is represented by the first six beats. 2. An atrial extrasystole. This occurs immediately after, and deforms the S-T segment of, the sixth beat. 3. Atrial fibrillation. The atrial extrasystole occurs very prematurely, i.e. during the vulnerable phase of the atria, and thus precipitates atrial fibrillation—the rest of the tracing. Note the chaotic baseline due to deformity by the *f* waves of the atrial fibrillation, and the irregular ventricular response.

SIGNIFICANCE

Atrial fibrillation occurs in mitral and tricuspid valvular disease, in coronary artery disease, thyrotoxicosis and in approximately 30 per cent of cases of constrictive pericarditis.

Paroxysmal atrial fibrillation occurs in the W-P-W syndrome (Chapter 19) and thyrotoxicosis.

Atrial fibrillation may occur in the absence of any other manifestation or organic heart disease and has been termed 'Lone Auricular Fibrillation' (Evans & Swann, 1954[1]). It usually occurs in young individuals who have no evidence of coronary artery disease. A familial incidence has also been reported. The phenomenon is probably due to the presence of an anomalous or additional A-V nodal by-pass congenital in origin—which permits rapid (reciprocal) return of the sinus impulse to the atria (Schamroth & Krikler, 1967[2]); a mechanism analogous to the Wolff-Parkinson-White syndrome (see Chapter 19). The rapidly returning impulse constitutes a source of very precipitate atrial fibrillation.

ATRIAL FLUTTER

Atrial flutter is the expression of a *rapid* and *regular* atrial excitation. This excitation may be due to two mechanisms either or both of which may be operative, viz.
1. *A circus movement* that results from a continuous, self-perpetuating circular path of excitation coursing around the orifices of the superior and inferior vena cavae.
2. *A focal discharge*—the rapid discharge of an ectopic atrial focus; similar to that of extrasystolic—paroxysmal—atrial tachycardia.

The ventricular response to this rapid atrial activity depends upon the efficacy of A-V conduction. Occasionally, every atrial impulse or excitatory circuit is conducted to the ventricles—a 1:1 response—resulting in a very fast ventricular rate (Fig. 130A). More commonly, second degree A-V block is present, e.g. in a ratio of 2:1, 4:1, 6:1 or 8:1, resulting in a relatively slow ventricular rate (Figs. 130—A II, B, C and D). Even ratios—2:1, 4:1 or 6:1—are commoner than odd ratios—3:1 or 5:1. Sometimes the conduction ratio fluctuates, e.g. from 4:1 to 6:1 to 2:1 ratios, etc.; this results in completely irregular ventricular rhythm. Regular 3:2 conduction ratios will result in ventricular bigeminal rhythm. Alternating 4:1 and 2:1 conduction ratios will also result in bigeminal rhythm (Fig. 184).

The flutter impulses may at times be conducted with phasic aberrant ventricular conduction (see Chapter 18 and Fig. 184).

ELECTROCARDIOGRAPHIC CHARACTERISTICS

The cardinal sign of atrial flutter is the presence of regular, undulating closely spaced but relatively wide atrial deflections or flutter—'F'—waves affecting the whole baseline and resulting in a *regular, corrugated or saw-tooth appearance* (Figs. 130 and 184). The isoelectric level between flutter waves is much shortened and is frequently not discernible. The T waves are usually masked or deformed by the flutter waves.

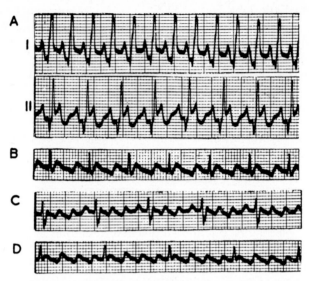

FIG. 130. Electrocardiograms (all tracings of Standard lead II) showing the various forms of flutter. (A) I shows atrial flutter with a 1:1 A-V response. (A) II is from the same patient after treatment with digitalis and shows a 2:1 A-V response. (B) shows atrial flutter with a 2:1 A-V response. (C) and (D) show atrial flutter with a 4:1 A-V response. Note (*a*) the rapid atrial rate; (*b*) the wide 'saw-tooth' deflections; (*c*) the absent or barely noticeable baseline.

Flutter waves are best seen in Standard lead II and lead VI. They are usually negative in Standard leads II and III, and lead AVF because the atrial activation tends to be directed caudo-cranially, i.e. a superiorly directed P or F wave axis.

The QRS complexes are normal unless there is coincidental bundle branch block, or a complicating phasic aberrant ventricular conduction (see Chapter 18 and Figs. 184 and 185).

When the saw-tooth appearance shows some irregularity or distortion suggestive of atrial fibrillation, the condition is sometimes referred to as *impure-flutter* or *flutter-fibrillation* (Fig. 131). It is doubtful, however, whether this represents a separate or finite entity; examples of this so-called condition are probably cases of uncomplicated atrial fibrillation.

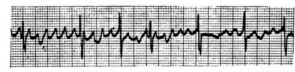

FIG. 131. Electrocardiogram illustrating so-called *flutter-fibrillation*.

Digitalis often converts atrial flutter to atrial fibrillation due to a shortening of the atrial refractory period. This may be followed by conversion to normal rhythm when the digitalis is stopped.

SIGNIFICANCE

Atrial flutter is commonly associated with chronic rheumatic valvular disease and ischaemic, hypertensive and pulmonary heart disease. Like paroxysmal atrial tachycardia, it has an abrupt onset and termination. The attacks of atrial flutter tend to last longer, however, and frequently precede permanent atrial fibrillation. Atrial flutter is more responsive to electrical cardioversion than any other tachyarrhythmia.

ATRIAL ESCAPE

(This is discussed in Chapter 14)

REFERENCES

1 EVANS W. & SWANN P. (1954) Lone auricular fibrillation. *Brit Heart J.* **16,** 189.
2 SCHAMROTH L. & KRIKLER D. M. (1967) The problem of lone atrial fibrillation. *S.A. Med. J.* **41,** 502.

CHAPTER 12

A-V Nodal Rhythms

THE CONDUCTION SEQUENCES OF A-V NODAL RHYTHMS

An impulse arising in the A-V node may have the following conduction sequences:

1. The nodal impulse may be conducted to the atria and ventricles (Fig. 132A, B and C).
2. The A-V nodal impulse may be conducted to the ventricles only, conduction to the atria being blocked or impeded by interference (Fig. 132D).
3. Occasionally, anterograde conduction of the A-V nodal impulse to the ventricles may be blocked or impeded by interference.

1. A-V NODAL RHYTHM WITH CONDUCTION TO ATRIA AND VENTRICLES

When the A-V nodal impulse is conducted to the atria and ventricles concomitantly, conduction to the ventricles usually proceeds along

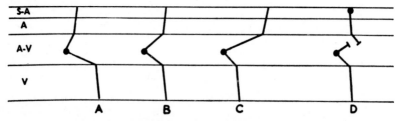

FIG. 132. Diagram illustrating various conduction mechanisms in A-V nodal rhythm (A) illustrates an A-V nodal beat with earlier retrograde conduction. (B) illustrates an A-V nodal beat with equal anterograde and retrograde conduction times. (C) illustrates an A-V nodal beat with late retrograde conduction. (D) illustrates an A-V nodal beat complicated by interference, resulting in a dissociated beat. The large black dots indicate impulse origin. S-A = sino-atrial level; A = atrial level; A-V = A-V nodal level; V = ventricular level.

normal A-V conduction pathways resulting in a normal QRST complex. Conduction to the atria, however, occurs retrogradely, i.e. the direction of atrial depolarization is reversed, and occurs from below upwards. As a result, *the P′ wave is inverted in leads where it is normally upright* and vice versa, i.e. it is inverted in Standard leads II and III, and lead AVF, upright in leads AVR and AVL, and usually equiphasic in Standard lead I (Fig. 135). In other words, the P′ wave vector is directed superiorly. The P′ wave is usually pointed and dominantly positive in lead VI. This contrasts with the normal diphasic sinus P wave.

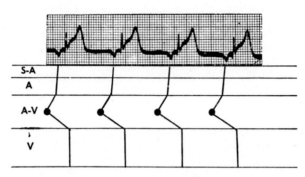

FIG. 133. Electrocardiogram (Standard lead II) showing A-V nodal rhythm with earlier retrograde conduction. An inverted P wave precedes each QRS complex. Large black dots indicate impulse origin.

RELATIONSHIP OF P WAVE TO QRS COMPLEX

Depending upon the relative velocity of anterograde and retrograde conduction, the P wave may *precede, follow, or occur synchronously with, and thus be hidden within, the QRS complex.*

(*a*) If retrograde conduction to the atria is relatively faster than anterograde conduction to the ventricles, the 'retrograde' P′ wave will *precede* the QRS complex; the P′–R interval is shortened (Figs. 132A and 133).

(*b*) If anterograde conduction to the ventricles is relatively faster than retrograde conduction to the atria the 'retrograde' P′ wave will *follow* the QRS complex (Figs. 132C, 134 and 135).

(*c*) If conduction to the atria and ventricles occurs at the same rate the 'retrograde' P′ wave will be recorded at the same time as, and be *hidden within*, the QRS complex (Fig. 132B).

2. A-V NODAL RHYTHM WITH CONDUCTION TO THE VENTRICLES ONLY

In this condition, conduction to the ventricles proceeds along normal pathways resulting in a normal QRST complex. Retrograde

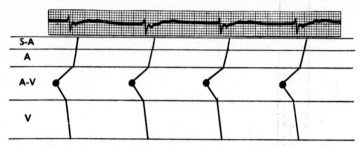

FIG. 134. Electrocardiogram (Standard lead II) showing A-V nodal rhythm with late retrograde conduction. *Note:* an inverted P wave follows each QRS complex. Large blacks dots indicate impulse origin.

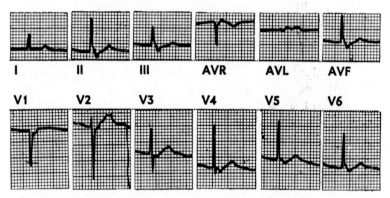

FIG. 135. Electrocardiogram showing A-V nodal rhythm with late retrograde conduction to, and activation of, the atria. Note (*a*) the P waves follow each QRS complex; (*b*) the P waves are inverted in Standard leads II and III and lead AVF.

conduction to the atria, however, does not occur, because of—

(*a*) a true retrograde block of the A-V nodal impulse (Fig. 195)

or

(*b*) interference with retrograde conduction of the A-V nodal impulse by a concomitant sinus impulse (Figs. 136, 155, 156 and 157).

In both these conditions, the sinus P waves are dissociated from the A-V nodal QRS complexes.

These manifestations of A-V nodal rhythm thus constitute a form of A-V dissociation (see section on A-V dissociation, Chapter 20).

THE FORMS OF A-V NODAL RHYTHM

A-V nodal rhythm may occur in the form of:

1. An **A-V nodal extrasystole** (Fig. 136).

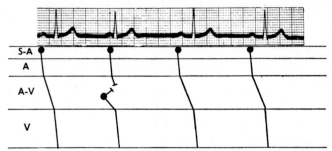

FIG. 136. Electrocardiogram showing an A-V nodal extrasystole. The first, third and fourth QRS complexes result from normal sinus beats conducted with first degree A-V block (P–R interval = 0.24 sec). The second QRS complex occurs prematurely and has virtually the same shape as the other QRS complexes; it is dissociated from the second sinus P wave. Black dots indicate impulse origin; S-A = sino-atrial level; A = atrial level; A-V = A-Vnodal level; V = ventricular level.

2. An **A-V nodal escape beat** (Figs. 155 and 157).
3. **Extrasystolic—paroxysmal—A-V nodal tachycardia** (Fig. 137).
4. **Idionodal tachycardia** (Fig. 138).

Note: The P-QRS relationship in all these A-V nodal rhythms may take any of the forms described above, viz. a 'retrograde' P wave is related to and may precede, follow, or be hidden within, the QRS complex; or a sinus P wave is unrelated to or dissociated from, the QRS complex.

1. A-V NODAL EXTRASYSTOLES

These have the same significance as atrial extrasystoles. If the A-V nodal extrasystole occurs with retrograde spread to the atria, the sinus node is usually discharged prematurely and the compensatory pause is incomplete. The sequence of events is similar to that occurring with an atrial extrasystole (see page 127).

If the A-V nodal extrasystole occurs without retrograde activation of the atria (Fig. 136), there is no interference with the sinus discharge, and the compensatory pause is complete. The sequence of events is similar to that occurring with most forms of ventricular extrasystoles (see page 148).

2. A-V NODAL ESCAPE BEAT

(This is discussed in Chapter 14)

3. EXTRASYSTOLIC—PAROXYSMAL—A-V NODAL TACHYCARDIA

This may be defined as a series of three or more A-V nodal extrasystoles (Fig. 137), and has the same significance as an atrial paroxysmal tachycardia.

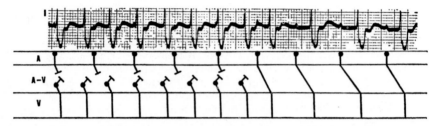

FIG. 137. Electrocardiogram (Standard lead I) showing: 1. Extra-systolic—paroxysmal—A-V nodal tachycardia, represented by the first eight QRS complexes. 2. A-V dissociation: the QRS complexes bear no relationship to the concomitant sinus rhythm; the P waves may be seen just before the QRS complexes or superimposed upon the S-T segments. 3. A ventricular capture beat. The 9th QRS complex is pre-mature and is related to the preceding P wave. This represents the con-duction to, and capture of, the ventricles by the preceding sinus impulse. 4. Sinus rhythm with first degree A-V block. The capture beat terminates the tachycardia, and sinus rhythm ensues. The P–R interval measures 0.22 sec. *Note*: (*a*) The QRS complexes of the conducted sinus impulses are identical to the QRS complexes of the ectopic tachycardia. This establishes the A-V nodal origin of the tachycardia, since the impulses of the tachycardia must have followed the same intraventricu-lar pathway as that used by the sinus impulses. (*b*) The sudden termina-tion of the ectopic tachycardia reflects its extrasystolic character.

IDIONODAL TACHYCARDIA
(Synonym: Non-paroxysmal A-V Nodal Tachycardia)

Idionodal tachycardia is the expression of an accelerated inherent idionodal rhythm, an enhancement of the inherent automaticity of a latent potential idionodal pacemaker—analogous to the enhancement of an idioventricular pacemaker in idioventricular tachycardia. The principles governing these arrhythmias are discussed in the section on idioventricular tachycardia (see page 156). The rhythm was first de-scribed by Pick & Dominguez (1957)[1] who termed it 'non-paroxysmal A-V nodal tachycardia' to distinguish it from the extrasystolic or paroxysmal forms of A-V nodal tachycardia.

ELECTROCARDIOGRAPHIC MANIFESTATIONS
The diagnosis of idionodal tachycardia is based on the following criteria:

1. CRITERIA FOR THE ESTABLISHMENT OF A-V NODAL ORIGIN
This is based upon:

A. The presence of a normal QRS complex or a QRS complex that has the same configuration as that of the conducted sinus impulse.
B. The conduction sequences characteristically associated with A-V nodal rhythms (see page 138).

2. AN ENHANCED IDIONODAL RATE
The normal inherent idionodal rate is usually in the range of 50 to 60 beats per minute. Allowing for some measure of overlap, an idionodal tachycardia may be arbitrarily defined as an idionodal rhythm whose rate exceeds 70 beats per minute. The rate of an idionodal tachycardia is most commonly between 70 and 100 beats per minute.

3. A PROPENSITY TO A-V DISSOCIATION
As the enhanced idionodal rhythm is usually in the same rate-range as that of the sinus rhythm, concomitant discharge is frequent, and A-V dissociation is therefore a common occurrence (Figs. 138 and 195).

4. A PROPENSITY TO VENTRICULAR CAPTURE BEATS
The relatively slow idionodal rate (when compared with the more rapid rates of extrasystolic A-V nodal tachycardia) results in a relatively long cycle length or diastolic period relative to the refractory period. This facilitates the opportunity for ventricular capture beats, since a sinus impulse that occurs during the end of the idionodal cycle will, under these circumstances, probably encounter responsive A-V nodal tissue, and be conducted to the ventricles. The rapid rate of the extra-systolic form of A-V nodal tachycardia results in a short cycle relative to the refractory period, and this militates against the occurrence of ventricular capture beats.

5. THE ABSENCE OF PACEMAKER PROTECTION
The absence of protection of the A-V nodal pacemaker in idionodal tachycardia is evident from:

A. The abolition of the idionodal tachycardia if and when the sinus rhythm accelerates and usurps control of the heart once again.
B. The 'dislocation' of the ectopic rhythm by a capture beat. The ectopic cycle is re-set by the capturing impulse, thereby indicating that the capturing impulse penetrated into the A-V nodal pacemaker site.

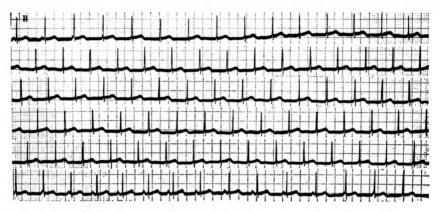

FIG. 138. The electrocardiogram (a continuous strip of Standard lead II) shows: 1. *Sinus rhythm*. This is evident at the beginning of the top strip and in the bottom strip where the P wave can be identified. The P–P intervals range from 0.60 sec to 0.70 sec reflecting a rate of 86 to 100 beats per minute—an expression of minimal sinus arrhythmia. 2. *Idionodal tachycardia*. This is reflected by the QRS complexes which are normal and bear no relationship to the P waves. The R–R intervals measure 0.64 sec representing a rate of 94 beats per minute. 3. *A-V dissociation*. The P waves and the QRS complexes are dissociated or unrelated. At the beginning of the recording, the P waves are seen to 'move into' the QRS complexes, i.e. the sinus rhythm attains the same rate as the idionodal rhythm. The two rhythms maintain this rate for about 45 seconds during which the P waves are hidden within the QRS complexes. The two rhythms become 'dislocated' once again in the bottom strip.

SIGNIFICANCE

The clinical significance of idionodal tachycardia is similar to that of idioventricular tachycardia (see page 158).

REFERENCE

1   PICK A. & DOMINGUEZ P. (1957) Nonparoxysmal A-V nodal tachycardia. *Circulation* **16**, 102.

CHAPTER 13

Ventricular Rhythms

VENTRICULAR EXTRASYSTOLES · VENTRICULAR
TACHYCARDIA · VENTRICULAR FLUTTER · VENTRICULAR
FIBRILLATION · VENTRICULAR PARASYSTOLE
VENTRICULAR ESCAPE

VENTRICULAR EXTRASYSTOLES

A ventricular extrasystole is due to the **premature** discharge of an
ectopic ventricular focus. It has the following characteristics:

1. THE DISCHARGE IS PREMATURE
The ventricular extrasystole is premature and arises in the diastolic
period of the preceding sinus beat. It is therefore recorded earlier than
the next anticipated sinus beat (Figs. 139, 140, 141, 142 and 143).

2. THE QRS COMPLEX IS BIZARRE
The discharge arises in an ectopic focus and the course of depolarization
is consequently abnormal. Furthermore, the impulse does not travel
through specialized conduction tissue but through ordinary muscle
tissue, which is a relatively poor conducting medium. As a result the
QRS complex is bizarre-widened and slurred or notched (Fig. 140).

3. SECONDARY S-T SEGMENT AND T WAVE CHANGES
The S-T segment may be depressed. The T wave is usually inverted
when the QRS complex is dominantly upright, and it is usually elevated
when the QRS complex is dominantly downward. These changes are
similar to those seen in classical right or left bundle branch block and
are secondary to the effects of abnormal depolarization.

4. THE COUPLING INTERVAL IS CONSTANT
The coupling interval is the interval between the ectopic beat and the
preceding sinus beat, and is constant for extrasystoles arising from the
same focus, i.e. extrasystoles of the same size and shape. This is because
the extrasystole is in some way related to, precipitated, or forced, by the
preceding sinus beat.

145

5. RELATIONSHIP TO THE FOLLOWING P WAVE

(A) *The ventricular extrasystoles may be dissociated from and have the following relationship to the ensuing sinus discharge:*

(i)   The extrasystole may discharge just before the following sinus discharge. When this occurs, the sinus P wave will be recorded after the bizarre QRS complex of the extrasystole and may be superimposed on the S-T segment of the extrasystole (Fig. 139).

(ii) The extrasystole may discharge at the same time as the following sinus discharge. When this occurs, the sinus P wave will be superimposed upon or hidden within the bizarre QRS complex of the extrasystole (Fig. 140).

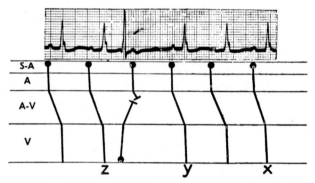

FIG. 139. Electrocardiogram showing a ventricular extrasystole which has discharged before the following sinus P wave. The P wave is recorded after the bizarre QRS complex and is seen superimposed on the S-T segment of the extrasystole. The compensatory pause is complete, i.e. the sum of the pre- and post-ectopic intervals (Z–Y) equals the sum of two consecutive sinus cycles (Y–X). Black dots indicate impulse origin.

(iii) The extrasystole may be discharged relatively late, i.e. just after the sinus discharge but before the sinus impulse reaches the ventricles (Fig. 141). The dissociated sinus P wave is then recorded just before the bizarre QRS complex of the extrasystole. The 'P–R' interval is very short. This is known as an *end-diastolic ventricular extrasystole.*

In all the instances cited above (Figs. 139, 140 and 141), the sinus and extrasystolic impulses meet and interfere with each other in the A–V node, i.e. the sinus impulse is prevented from passing to the ventricles, and the ventricular impulse is prevented from passing to the atria.

(B) *Retrograde conduction of the ventricular extrasystole*

Occasionally, in the presence of a basic sinus bradycardia, or when the

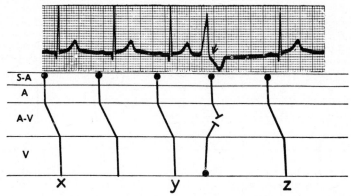

FIG. 140. Electrocardiogram (Standard lead II) showing a ventricular extrasystole. Note (*a*) the bizarre premature QRS complex of the extrasystole which occurs concomitantly with a sinus discharge; the P wave of this sinus discharge is thus largely hidden within the QRST complex of the extrasystole but may just be seen as a slight deformity (barely discernible) on the proximal part of the S-T segment (arrow); (*b*) the compensatory pause is complete, i.e. the sum of the pre- and post-ectopic intervals (Y–Z) is exactly equal to two consecutive sinus cycles (X–Y)—(see also Fig. 139).

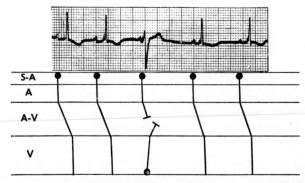

FIG. 141. Electrocardiogram (Standard lead II) showing a ventricular extrasystole which has discharged relatively late—an end-diastolic ventricular extrasystole, i.e. it occurs just after the following sinus discharge. The P wave of this sinus discharge is thus recorded just before the bizarre complex of the ventricular extrasystole (see also Fig. 144A).

ventricular extrasystole is very premature, the extrasystolic discharge occurs long before the next scheduled sinus discharge. Consequently, the ectopic impulse reaches the A-V node and atria *before* they have been activated by the sinus impulse. The ectopic impulse can then be conducted retrogradely to the atria and may even reach the S-A node

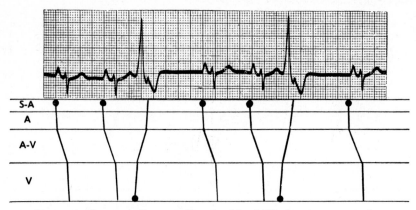

FIG. 142. Electrocardiogram (Standard lead II) showing ventricular extrasystoles with retrograde conduction to the atria. Note (a) an inverted P wave follows each extrasystole; (b) the inverted P wave is premature, i.e. it occurs earlier than the next anticipated sinus P wave (the normal P–P interval = 0.80 sec, the interval between the inverted P wave and the preceding P wave = 0.68 sec). Large black dots indicate impulse origin.

and discharge it prematurely (Fig. 142). The bizarre QRS complex of the ventricular extrasystole is thus followed by a premature and 'retrograde'—usually inverted—P wave (compare A-V nodal extrasystoles with retrograde conduction—page 141). See also section on Interpolated Ventricular Extrasystoles (page 149).

6. THE COMPENSATORY PAUSE

When the ventricular extrasystole is dissociated from the sinus impulse (described above in paragraphs 5 (i), (ii), (iii)), the ectopic impulse is unable to penetrate the A-V node retrogradely. The discharge of the

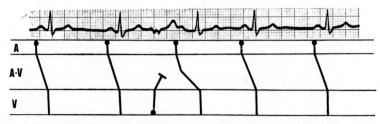

FIG. 143. Electrocardiogram showing an interpolated ventricular extrasystole. Note (a) the ventricular extrasystole is 'sandwiched' between two sinus beats; (b) there is no disturbance of sinus rhythm; (c) the P–R interval of the sinus beat following the extrasystole is longer than the P–R interval of the sinus beat preceding the extrasystole. Black dots indicate impulse origin.

S-A node is thus not interfered with and the S-A node is, in a sense, protected from the ectopic impulse. The sinus rhythm continues undisturbed, i.e. the next sinus impulse (the one following the dissociated beat) occurs on schedule. The pause following the extrasystole—the compensatory pause—is thus complete, i.e. it compensates exactly for the extrasystolic prematurity—the sum of the pre- and post-ectopic intervals (Y–Z in Figs. 139 and 140) is exactly equal to the sum of two consecutive sinus intervals (X–Y in Figs. 139 and 140).

With retrograde conduction of the ventricular extrasystole (described in (B) above), the sinus node is discharged prematurely by the ectopic impulse and the compensatory pause is consequently incomplete (compare sequence of events in atrial extrasystole—page 127).

7. THE 'RULE OF BIGEMINY'

Ventricular extrasystoles tend to follow long R–R intervals—the 'Rule of Bigeminy' (Langendorf, Pick & Winternitz, 1955[1]). This phenomenon is best seen during irregular rhythms, e.g. marked sinus arrhythmia or atrial fibrillation (Fig. 145). The compensatory pause of the extrasystole in turn, constitutes another long R–R interval which tends to precipitate a further extrasystole. This process is thus self-perpetuating resulting in bigeminal rhythm.

INTERPOLATED VENTRICULAR EXTRASYSTOLES

An interpolated ventricular extrasystole is an extrasystole which is, so-to-speak, 'sandwiched' between two conducted sinus beats (Fig. 143). It therefore occurs without a compensatory pause. Interpolated ventricular extrasystoles are usually associated with slow sinus rhythms.

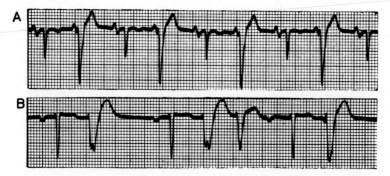

FIG. 144. Electrocardiograms (both tracings of lead V1) showing bigeminal rhythm due to alternate ventricular extrasystoles. (A) shows end-diastolic ventricular extrasystoles (compare Fig. 141). Note the constant coupling intervals. (B) shows an instance of ventricular trigeminy resulting from a pair of consecutive ventricular extrasystoles.

MECHANISM

(a) The ventricular extrasystole occurs very early, i.e. at a time when the A-V node is still refractory; retrograde conduction of the ectopic impulse to the atria is therefore blocked within the A-V node.

(b) The following sinus beat occurs on time, but relatively late to the extrasystole; it thus finds the A-V node and ventricles sufficiently recovered to respond; nevertheless, owing to some retrograde penetration of the ectopic impulse into the A-V node, the lower, or penetrated, region of the A-V node is still a little refractory, and the following sinus beat is therefore conducted with delay, resulting in a longer than usual P–R interval.

CHARACTERISTICS OF INTERPOLATED VENTRICULAR EXTRASYSTOLES

1. They occur during slow sinus rhythm.
2. The extrasystole is 'sandwiched' between two sinus beats and there is no compensatory pause.
3. The sinus beat following the extrasystole has a longer P–R interval than the sinus beat preceding the extrasystole.

EXTRASYSTOLIC VENTRICULAR BIGEMINY

Alternate ventricular extrasystoles, i.e. extrasystoles which occur after every other sinus beat, are the commonest cause of bigeminal rhythm (Fig. 144) and a frequent manifestation of digitalis intoxication.

MULTIFOCAL OR MULTIFORM VENTRICULAR EXTRASYSTOLES

Extrasystoles that arise from different foci and consequently give rise to different QRS complexes are termed multifocal or multiform ventricular extrasystoles (Fig. 145).

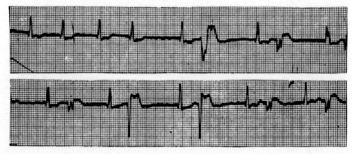

FIG. 145. Electrocardiogram (continuous strip of Standard lead II) showing (a) atrial fibrillation; (b) multiform ventricular extrasystoles. Note the first ventricular extrasystole follows a long R–R interval—the 'Rule of Bigeminy'.

EXTRASYSTOLES IN PAIRS

When a ventricular ectopic focus discharges prematurely and twice in succession, the rhythm will manifest as a pair of extrasystoles, viz. a sinus beat followed by two extrasystoles (Figs. 144 and 146C).

EXTRASYSTOLIC—PAROXYSMAL—VENTRICULAR TACHYCARDIA

Three or more successive ventricular extrasystoles constitute an extra-systolic ventricular tachycardia—a paroxysmal tachycardia (Fig. 146).

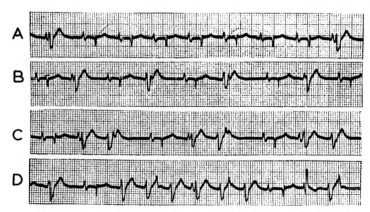

FIG. 146. Electrocardiograms illustrating various levels of ectopic ventricular irritability. A = occasional ventricular extrasystoles. B = extrasystoles in bigeminal rhythm. C = extrasystoles in pairs. D = paroxysmal ventricular tachycardia.

SIGNIFICANCE OF VENTRICULAR EXTRASYSTOLES

Although isolated ventricular extrasystoles may occasionally be found in a normal individual, their presence should always be viewed with suspicion.

Ventricular extrasystoles are always significant when associated with myocardial disease.

Multifocal ventricular extrasystoles and ventricular extrasystoles in pairs are *always* abnormal and usually indicative of serious myocardial disease.

Unifocal ventricular extrasystoles are usually indicative of cardiac disease if (*a*) they occur frequently, i.e. in 'crops' or 'showers', (*b*) they occur in bigeminal rhythm, (*c*) they occur in association with cardiac disease, (*d*) they occur in persons over 40 years of age, (*e*) they are precipitated by exercise.

Frequent ventricular extrasystoles, especially those occurring in pairs, often herald ventricular tachycardia or ventricular fibrillation.

The following schema is a rough but not necessarily absolute guide to the state of ectopic ventricular automaticity.

In the early stages of ectopic ventricular irritability, only occasional extrasystoles are evident (Fig. 146, strip A). Further evolution, i.e. increasing ventricular automaticity, is manifested by (a) ventricular extrasystoles in bigeminal rhythm (strip B), (b) extrasystoles in pairs (strip C) and (c) ventricular tachycardia (strip D).

Ventricular extrasystoles complicating myocardial infarction worsen the prognosis.

Digitalis intoxication is the commonest cause of ventricular extrasystolic bigeminal rhythm and the advent of this rhythm during digitalis administration is an absolute indication to stop therapy. Digitalis intoxication will rarely, if ever, cause ventricular extrasystolic bigeminal rhythm in a normal heart.

VENTRICULAR EXTRASYSTOLES WITH VERY SHORT COUPLING INTERVALS: THE 'R ON T' PHENOMENON

A ventricular extrasystole may rarely occur with a very short coupling interval, and will consequently coincide with, and be superimposed upon, or near, the apex or the distal limb of the preceding T wave (Fig. 154). Ventricular extrasystoles with this marked prematurity reflect an ominous situation for they are then likely to occur during the 'vulnerable phase' of the recovering ventricular myocardium and will consequently be prone to precipitate ventricular fibrillation.

VENTRICULAR TACHYCARDIA

Ventricular tachycardia is due to the rapid discharge of an ectopic ventricular pacemaking focus. It may be defined as a series of three or more consecutive ventricular ectopic beats which are recorded in rapid succession. There are two principal forms:

1. **Extrasystolic Ventricular Tachycardia.**
2. **Idioventricular Tachycardia.**

EXTRASYSTOLIC VENTRICULAR TACHYCARDIA

Extrasystolic ventricular tachycardia is a series of three or more consecutive ventricular extrasystoles.

ELECTROCARDIOGRAPHIC MANIFESTATIONS

1. BIZARRE QRS COMPLEXES

The QRS complexes have the characteristics of ventricular extra-systoles, i.e. they are bizarre, premature, and are recorded in rapid succession (Figs. 146, 147 and 148).

2. A-V DISSOCIATION

The ectopic ventricular rhythm and the sinus rhythm may be dissociated. When this occurs, the sinus impulses and the ectopic ventricular

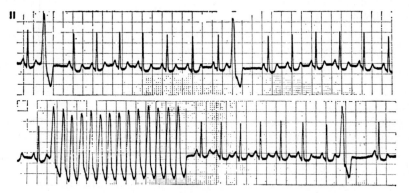

FIG. 147. Electrocardiogram (continuous strip of Standard lead II) showing: 1. Sinus tachycardia, reflected by the normal P-QRS-T complexes recorded in rapid succession; rate = 120 beats per minute. 2. Ventricular extrasystoles, reflected by the bizarre, isolated, and premature QRS complexes. A paroxysm of extrasystolic ventricular tachycardia, reflected by the series of 14 consecutive ventricular extrasystoles recorded in very rapid succession.

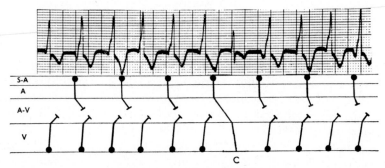

FIG. 148. Electrocardiogram illustrating paroxysmal ventricular tachycardia. Note (a) the bizarre QRS complexes of the ectopic discharge which are completely dissociated from the P waves of the sinus discharge; (b) the complex labelled C represents a capture beat—it is near-normal in configuration and is preceded by a P wave (seen superimposed on the preceding T wave).

impulses meet within the A-V node and impede or interfere with each other's mutual progress (compare with the dissociated form of ventricular extrasystoles—Section A on page 146). The **P waves therefore bear no relationship to the QRS complexes** (Figs. 146, 147 and 148).

3. RETROGRADE V-A CONDUCTION

The ectopic ventricular impulses may, at times, be conducted retrogradely to the atria (Fig. 181). Activation of the atria is then effected retrogradely by the ectopic ventricular impulses, and the bizarre QRS complexes are then followed by 'retrograde' P' waves: P' waves which are inverted in Standard leads II and III, and lead AVF, and which are pointed and dominantly positive in lead V1.

Note: Every QRS complex is followed by an abnormal P' wave but it is often difficult, and at times impossible, to tell (*a*) whether such P' waves are the result of ventricular tachycardia with retrograde conduction, or (*b*) whether they represent atrial paroxysmal tachycardia with phasic aberrant ventricular conduction (see page 186). The diagnosis can only be made with certainty when the beginning of a paroxysm is recorded: in the case of a ventricular tachycardia, the abnormal P' wave will *follow* the first bizarre QRS complex, whereas in atrial paroxysmal tachycardia with phasic aberrant ventricular conduction, the abnormal P' wave will *precede* the first bizarre QRS complex (Fig. 180).

4. CAPTURE BEATS

When the sinus rhythm and the ventricular rhythm are dissociated, their impulses meet and interfere with each other's mutual progress within the A-V node. In other words, the A-V node is in a state of almost constant refractoriness due to prior penetration by either the sinus or ectopic impulses. Occasionally, however, with critical timing, and especially during relatively slow ventricular tachycardias, a sinus impulse may reach the A-V node during a non-refractory phase, i.e. just after a period of absolute refractoriness following partial retrograde penetration of the ectopic impulse into the A-V node. The sinus impulse can then be conducted to the ventricles and momentarily activate or capture the ventricles, i.e. for one beat only (Fig. 148). This conducted beat which occurs during the ectopic ventricular rhythm is known as a *capture beat*. The QRS complex of the capture beat is recognized because it resembles the conducted sinus beats during regular sinus rhythm. Furthermore, the capture beat is always related to a preceding sinus P wave (see also section on interference-dissociation—page 204). A capture beat whose configuration differs from the QRS configuration of the basic ventricular tachycardia, is one of the more reliable diagnostic pointers to the ventricular origin of the basic tachycardia.

5. VENTRICULAR FUSION

At times, the capturing (sinus) impulse may invade the ventricles concomitantly with the ectopic ventricular impulse. When this occurs, each impulse will activate part of the ventricles, and the resulting QRS complex will have a configuration that is in between that of the 'pure' sinus beat (seen during uncomplicated sinus rhythm) and the 'pure' ectopic

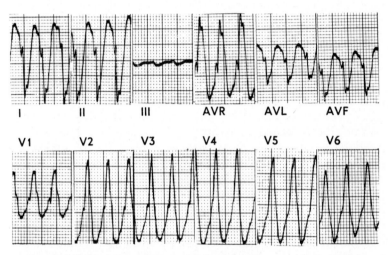

FIG. 149. The P waves and the P : QRS relationship cannot be accurately identified. The electrocardiogram nevertheless reflects the following features which indicate a diagnosis of extrasystolic ventricular tachycardia. 1. The mean manifest frontal plane axis is directed at −150°. This is a bizarre and unusual axis. In the case of phasic aberrant ventricular conduction the axis would tend to be normally directed. 2. The QRS complexes do not resemble the typical forms of either left or right bundle branch block. 3. The horizontal plane leads reflect the *concordant pattern*; the QRS complexes are upright in *all* the precordial leads.

beat. This combination or summation beat is known as a *ventricular fusion beat* (see also section on ventricular fusion beats in ventricular parasystole—page 210). A ventricular fusion beat is the most reliable diagnostic pointer to the ventricular origin of the basic tachycardia.

SIGNIFICANCE

Extrasystolic—paroxysmal—ventricular tachycardia is usually associated with advanced myocardial disease, most commonly ischaemic heart disease, and is frequently a manifestation of digitalis intoxication.

IDIOVENTRICULAR TACHYCARDIA

The heart has many potential pacemaking cells which are situated in the S-A node, the atria, the A-V node, and the ventricles. Only one of these pacemaking cells—the pacemaker with the highest automaticity or discharge rate—is, however, in control of the heart. This is because its impulses reach the slower potential subsidiary pacemakers, and abolish or discharge their immature impulses before they have the time or opportunity to reach maturity and 'fire'. The subsidiary pacemaking centres thus enjoy *no protection* from the impulses of the fastest pacemaker; and it is this which ensures that only one pacemaker is normally in control of the heart.

The inherent automaticity of the S-A node and the potential subsidiary pacemakers may, under certain circumstances, become enhanced. When, for example, the inherent automaticity of the S-A node is enhanced, the rhythm manifests as a sinus tachycardia. The inherent rate of the A-V nodal pacemaker—the idionodal rhythm—may be similarly enhanced, and if the enhanced A-V nodal rate exceeds the sinus rate, the A-V nodal rhythm becomes manifest. This accelerated idionodal rhythm is known as *idionodal tachycardia*. An inherent idioventricular rhythm may be similarly enhanced resulting in an *idioventricular tachycardia*.

If an enhanced idionodal rhythm or an enhanced idioventricular rhythm is to become manifest, it is clear that a disproportionate or differential enhancing influence must be present; an influence that affects the idionodal rhythm or the idioventricular rhythm to a greater degree than the sinus rhythm, or, an influence that only affects a particular pacemaker.

ELECTROCARDIOGRAPHIC CRITERIA

The diagnosis of idioventricular tachycardia is based on the following manifestations (Figs. 151 and 152):

1. Evidence of ventricular origin, e.g. bizarre QRS complexes, ventricular fusion beats (see also page 188).
2. A *relatively* rapid idioventricular rate. The idioventricular rhythm is usually accelerated to the same rate-range as that of the sinus rhythm, i.e. in the range of 70 to 80 beats per minute.
3. *A propensity to A-V dissociation and capture beats.* Since idioventricular tachycardia usually occurs in approximately the same rate-range as that of sinus rhythm, the two rhythms commonly discharge simultaneously (Fig. 150). A-V dissociation is therefore a common occurrence. Furthermore, capture beats—both complete and incomplete (fusion beats)—are also very common. This is due to the *relatively* slow rate of the idioventricular tachycardia; the relatively

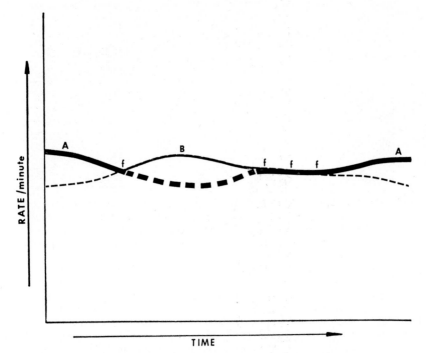

RATE/minute

TIME

FIG. 150. Diagram illustrating the mechanism of idioventricular tachycardia. The idioventricular rhythm (B) is enhanced to the same rate of the sinus rhythm (A). Slight fluctuation in the rate of these rhythms results in one and then the other becoming dominant and manifest. Transition from one rhythm to the other is marked by fusion beats (f). Since the rates of both rhythms may, at times, be fortuitously synchronous, there may be periods with consecutive fusion beats (f f f).

long cycle permits adequate recovery time, and thereby a greater opportunity for capture. With very fast rates, as occurs in extrasystolic ventricular tachycardia, the refractory period frequently occupies the whole or practically the whole ectopic cycle, and the opportunity for capture is consequently minimal or absent.

Since idioventricular tachycardia becomes manifest when its rate equals the sinus rate, the ectopic rhythm usually begins with several consecutive fusion beats—incomplete capture beats (Fig. 151). And since the two rhythms tend to fluctuate within the same narrow range, the ectopic rhythm tends to terminate with several successive fusion complexes.

4. *The absence of pacemaker protection.* The ectopic pacemaker has no protection. This is evident from the abolition of the ectopic rhythm if and when the sinus rhythm regains its dominance. This is in contrast

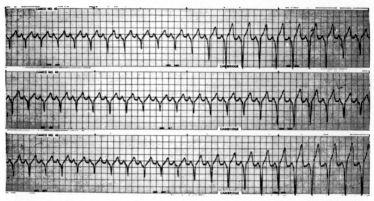

FIG. 151. The electrocardiogram (a continuous recording of Standard lead II) was recorded from a 66-year-old man with acute inferior myocardial infarction, and shows: 1. *Sinus tachycardia*. The P–P intervals measure 0.56 sec reflecting a rate of 107 beats per minute. 2. *Idioventricular tachycardia*. This is represented by the bizarre QRS complexes at the end of each strip. These bizarre QRS complexes are not related to the P waves which occur just before, and are sometimes superimposed upon or hidden within, the proximal part of the bizarre QRS complexes. This reflects the presence of A-V dissociation. The R–R intervals measure 0.56 sec representing a rate of 107 beats per minute— a ventricular tachycardia. The 'pure' ectopic complex is represented, for example, by the seven bizarre QRS complexes at the end of the top strip. The two QRS complexes preceding and the two QRS complexes following this period of idioventricular tachycardia have a configuration that is in between that of the 'pure' ectopic beat and the 'pure' sinus beat. These are ventricular fusion complexes. Every period of ectopic ventricular rhythm begins and ends with ventricular fusion complexes. Ventricular fusion complexes may also be seen during the periods of dominant sinus rhythm, e.g. the 6th, 7th and 8th QRS complexes in the top strip are slightly modified, reflecting partial ventricular fusion.

to ventricular parasystole where the ectopic rhythm is never abolished by a faster sinus rhythm (see page 208).

SIGNIFICANCE

Idioventricular tachycardia is the expression of *non-specific enhancement* of a pacemaker, and may, for example, be associated with such non-specific 'activity' as *fever* and carditis. It is not infrequently associated with the administration of digitalis and is a common manifestation in acute myocardial infarction; commoner, in fact, than extrasystolic ventricular tachycardia.

As with sinus tachycardia, the rhythm itself rarely requires any active treatment. It is not a sudden precipitous, dramatic event, and is unlikely to precipitate ventricular fibrillation. Since it is usually in the

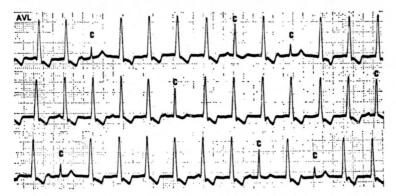

F IG. 152. Electrocardiogram (lead AVL) showing *idioventricular tachy-cardia*. This is reflected by the bizarre QRS complexes which are re-corded at a rate of 104 beats per minute, and which bear no relation-ship to the P waves of the sinus rhythm. The rhythm is complicated by frequent capture beats (labelled C): the momentary conduction to, and capture of, the ventricles by the sinus impulse. Some of these capture beats are incomplete, i.e. the sinus impulse invades the ventricles con-comitantly with the ventricular impulse, each activating part of the ven-tricles. This results in a ventricular fusion complex, a complex whose configuration is in between that of the 'pure' sinus beat and the 'pure' ectopic beat. The configuration of these partial capture beats varies and depends upon the relative contribution of each impulse to ventricular activation. When the contribution from the ectopic ventricular impulse is dominant, the ventricular fusion complex resembles the 'pure' ectopic beat, e.g. eighth QRS complex in the top strip and the last QRS complex in the middle strip. When the contribution from the sinus impulse is greater, the QRS complex will tend to resemble the 'pure' sinus beat, e.g. the third and tenth complexes in the top strip, and the second and eleventh QRS complexes in the bottom strip.

same rate-range as that of the normal sinus rhythm, it rarely causes haemodynamic embarrassment. If the loss of atrial drive becomes significant (a rare event) the ectopic ventricular rhythm may be over-driven by accelerating the sinus rate with atropine. It is doubtful whether it is ever necessary to resort to electrical overdriving or the use of cardio-suppressive drugs such as lidocaine.

VENTRICULAR FLUTTER

Ventricular flutter is the expression of:

1. *A very rapid and regular ectopic ventricular discharge.*

2. *Grossly abnormal intraventricular conduction.* The QRS and T deflec-tions are very wide and bizarre—one merging with the other—so that it is difficult to define or separate the QRS complex, S-T segment and T

wave. This results in the appearance of a continuous sine-like wave-form (Fig. 153).

Note: This bizarre sine-like wave-form may result from the abnormal intraventricular conduction alone. The appearance of ventricular flutter may thus occur at rates similar to that of extrasystolic ventricular tachycardia.

Co-ordinated activation and consequent haemodynamic contraction is still present. However, the change from extrasystolic tachycardia to ventricular flutter is associated with a fall in blood pressure and cardiac output (Smirk, Nolla-Panades & Wallis, 1964[2]).

Ventricular flutter is uncommon. Few examples are recorded since the condition usually progresses or changes rapidly to ventricular fibrillation.

Ventricular flutter differs from ventricular fibrillation by the uniformity, constancy, regularity, and relatively large amplitude of the deflections. The deflections of ventricular fibrillation are small and completely chaotic and irregular.

It may well be that ventricular flutter and extrasystolic ventricular tachycardia are expressions of the same mechanism. Their separation

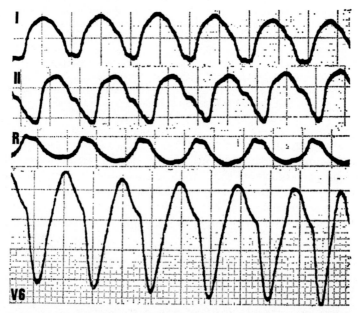

FIG. 153. Electrocardiogram showing ventricular flutter. The QRS complexes are very wide, bizarre, and blend imperceptibly with the T waves so that a separation of the two is difficult. The effect is that of a continuous 'sine-like' wave form (best seen in Standard lead I).

may, nevertheless, serve a useful purpose, since a diagnosis of ventricular flutter immediately connotes a very rapid ventricular rate and/or grossly abnormal intraventricular conduction, and reflects an ominous clinical state with a drop in blood pressure and a low cardiac output.

VENTRICULAR FIBRILLATION

Ventricular fibrillation is usually a terminal event. The electrocardiogram manifests with *completely irregular, chaotic and deformed deflections* of varying height, width and shape (Fig. 154).

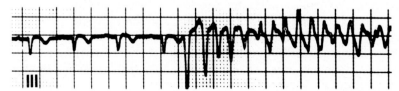

FIG. 154. Electrocardiogram showing sinus rhythm for the first 4 beats. These beats reflect the fully evolved phase of inferior wall myocardial infarction. The fourth beat is followed by a very premature ventricular extrasystole which occurs near the apex of the T wave of the sinus beat —the 'R on T' phenomenon. This precipitates ventricular fibrillation. Note the complete irregularity in the size, shape and rhythm of the electrocardiographic deflection. There is no recognizable pattern.

SIGNIFICANCE

Ventricular fibrillation is usually associated with advanced ischaemic heart disease. It may occur as a complication of complete A-V block and cardiac surgery, and may follow the administration of digitalis, adrenaline and anaesthetics.

VENTRICULAR PARASYSTOLE

(This is discussed in Chapter 21)

VENTRICULAR ESCAPE

(This is discussed in Chapter 14)

REFERENCES

1 LANGENDORF R., PICK A. & WINTERNITZ M. (1955) Mechanisms of intermittent ventricular bigeminy. *Circulation* **11,** 422.
2 SMIRK F. H., NOLLA-PANADES J. & WALLIS T. (1964) Experimental ventricular flutter and paroxysmal tachycardia. *Amer. J. Cardiol.* **14,** 79.

Escape Rhythms

The heart has many potential pacemakers which are situated in the sino-atrial node, the atria, the A-V node, and the ventricles. Each pacemaker has its own inherent rate and cycle length. The more distal the pacemaker is situated from the S-A node, the slower its automaticity or inherent discharge rate. However, it is only the fastest pacemaker—the pacemaker with the highest automaticity (usually the S-A node)—that is normally in control in the heart, since its impulses reach the slower subsidiary pacemakers before they have an opportunity to 'fire' and discharge or abolish their immature impulses prematurely. The cycle of the subsidiary pacemaker must then begin anew, i.e. from the moment of its passive discharge by the faster pacemaker. This reset ectopic cycle will again be interrupted by the next sinus impulse. At times, however, the impulses from the fastest pacemaker fail to reach the slower subsidiary pacemaker. When this occurs, the impulses from a slower subsidiary pacemaker (in the atria, A-V node or ventricles) have an opportunity to reach maturity and are thus able to discharge spon-

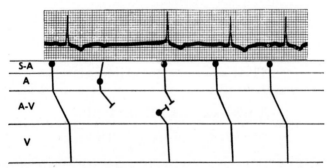

Fig. 155. Electrocardiogram showing A-V nodal escape following a blocked atrial extrasystole. Note (*a*) the QRS complex following the blocked atrial extrasystole is normal in shape and is not preceded by a P wave; (*b*) the sinus discharge following the extrasystole occurs synchronously with the A-V nodal discharge and is therefore hidden within the A-V nodal QRS complex.

taneously. This spontaneous discharge of a slower subsidiary pacemaker is known as an *escape beat* (Figs. 155 and 158), since the slower pacemaker has so to speak 'escaped' from the influence of the faster pacemaker. If the subsidiary pacemaker is able to discharge from two or more beats, the rhythm is known as *escape rhythm* (Figs. 156 and 157).

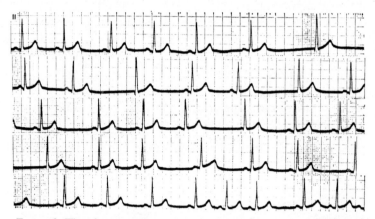

FIG. 156. The electrocardiogram (a continuous strip of Standard lead II) shows: 1. *Sinus rhythm with sinus arrhythmia and periods of sinus brady-cardia.* 2. *A-V nodal escape.* The long pauses resulting from the sinus bradycardia are terminated by A-V nodal escape beats. These escape beats are represented by the last QRS complex in the top strip, the third and sixth QRS complexes in the second strip, the second and fifth QRS complexes in the third strip, and the first QRS complex in the fourth strip. These escape beats have QRS complexes of identical contour to those of the conducted sinus beats. The near synchronous P waves of the sinus rhythm are dissociated from the QRS complexes and are superimposed upon the QRS complexes of the escape beats, or occur just before the escape beats with a shorter 'P–R' interval.

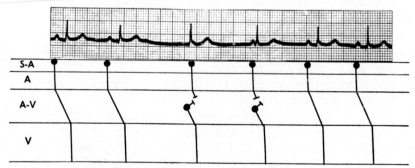

FIG. 157. Electrocardiogram showing two A-V nodal escape beats following S-A block—the result of marked sinus arrhythmia. Black dots indicate impulse origin. S-A = sino-atrial level; A = atrial level; A-V = A-V nodal level; V = ventricular level.

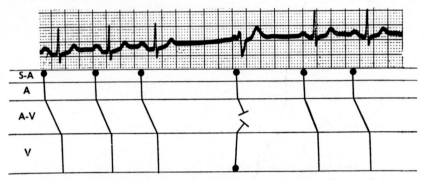

FIG. 158. Electrocardiogram showing ventricular escape following S-A block. Note (*a*) the bizarre QRS complex occurs late and follows a pause; (*b*) the ectopic discharge occurs near-synchronously with the sinus discharge resulting in a dissociated beat; (*c*) the P–R interval of conducted beats is prolonged (0.23 sec).

Basic Causes

Failure of sinus impulses to reach the slower subsidiary pacemaker may be due to two basic disturbances:

A. *Primary depression of the sinus pacemaker.* This is a depression or slowing of impulse formation as represented by sinus bradycardia.

B. *Conduction failure of the sinus impulses.* Failure of the faster sinus impulses to reach the slower subsidiary pacemaker may also be due to a conduction disturbance which prevents the sinus impulse from reaching the slower subsidiary pacemaker, e.g. S-A block and second or third degree A-V block (Figs. 167 to 171).

Thus, escape rhythm is a *consequence of* primary failure of the sinus rhythm, and, as such, is never a primary diagnosis.

Electrocardiographic Manifestations

1. The escape beat occurs *late*, i.e. it follows an interval that is longer than the dominant cycle length.
2. Atrial escape is characterized by the late inscription of an abnormal P wave—a P′ deflection (Fig. 159).
3. A-V nodal escape is characterized by the late inscription of an A-V nodal beat (Figs. 155, 156 and 157).
4. Ventricular escape is characterized by the late inscription of a bizarre QRS complex of a ventricular beat (Fig. 158).

SIGNIFICANCE

Escape beats only occur as a result of primary pacemaker default. They

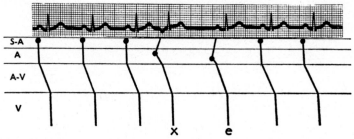

FIG. 159. Electrocardiogram illustrating (*a*) normal sinus rhythm—first three P-QRS-T complexes; (*b*) an atrial extrasystole—beat labelled x; note the premature and bizarre P wave; (*c*) an atrial escape beat—labelled e; note the *late* P wave of different contour than the normal sinus P wave.

are therefore a secondary phenomenon, and do not have any primary significance. Thus, the significance of escape rhythm is the significance of the sinus bradycardia, S-A block or A-V block which leads to the escape. Escape rhythm is never a primary diagnosis.

CHAPTER 15

Electrical Alternans

Electrical alternans is an electrocardiographic manifestation in which there is alternation in the amplitude of the QRS complexes and occasionally the T waves (Fig. 160). It often accompanies fast rates and then has no prognostic significance. When found with slow rates it has the same significance as its mechanical counterpart and usually connotes organic heart disease with an adverse prognosis.

Note: Electrical alternans does not cause a disturbance of rhythm.

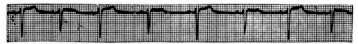

Fig. 160. Electrocardiogram showing electrical alternans. Note (*a*) the alternation in the amplitude of the QRS complexes and T waves; (*b*) there is no disturbance of rhythm. This electrical alternans is significant as it occurs with a relatively slow heart rate.

Disorders of Impulse Conduction

S-A BLOCK · A-V BLOCK · PHASIC ABERRANT
VENTRICULAR CONDUCTION

CHAPTER 16

Sino-Atrial (S-A) Block

In S-A block the sinus impulse is blocked *within* the S-A junction, i.e. the junction between the S-A node and the surrounding atrial myocardium. As a result, neither atrial nor ventricular activation takes place; no P wave or QRS complex is recorded, i.e. a *complete cardiac cycle 'drops out'* (Fig. 161). This may occur irregularly and unpredictably in isolated

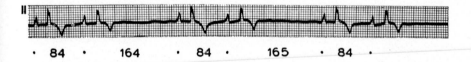

· 84 · 164 · 84 · 165 · 84 ·

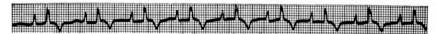

FIG. 161. *Top strip*: Electrocardiogram (Standard lead II) showing:
1. First degree A-V block. The P–R intervals measure 0.25 sec. 2. 3:2 S-A block. The P waves are distributed in a bigeminal grouping of long and short intervals. The relatively short P–P intervals of 0.84 sec alternate with intervals of 1.65 sec—almost twice the cycle length of the shorter interval. This indicates that the long interval is due to the omission of a complete P-QRS complex. Every third sinus impulse is blocked at the S-A junction resulting in a 3:2 S-A block. This causes a bigeminal rhythm.
   Bottom strip: This was recorded after the administration of atropine. The S-A block is abolished and this is associated with a slight increase in the sinus rate.

167

instances. Very rarely, the block may occur at regular intervals, e.g. regular 2:1 S-A block. This resembles the slow regular rhythm of sinus bradycardia; the diagnosis can only be established when, in contrast to the gradual acceleration of sinus bradycardia, the rate suddenly doubles with effort or atropine.

Following S-A block, the subsequent beat may be a normal sinus beat (Fig. 161), an A-V nodal escape beat (Fig. 157), or a ventricular escape beat (Fig. 158).

N te: In S-A block, *neither* the P wave *nor* the QRS complex is recorded at the moment of block; whereas in 2nd degree A-V block, *all* P waves are recorded; the P wave of the blocked beat is *not* followed by a QRS complex.

SIGNIFICANCE

S-A block is found in the same conditions as marked sinus bradycardia or sinus arrhythmia. It occurs in young vagotonic individuals, particularly athletes, and also with digitalis administration. It is not infrequently associated with uraemia and occasionally with hypokalaemia.

Atrioventricular (A-V) Block

Atrioventricular (A-V) block is characterized by a delay **or interruption in conduction** of the atrial impulse through the specialized A-V conducting system: the A-V node and the bundle of His.
There are three grades or degrees:

1. **First degree A-V block:** a delay in conduction.
2. **Second degree A-V block:** intermittent interruption of conduction.
3. **Third degree A-V block:** complete or permanent interruption of conduction.

First and second degree A-V block are often referred to as *partial* or *incomplete A-V block*. A-V block is often loosely called heart block. This term, however, has a wider meaning and embraces all forms of heart block, viz. sino-atrial block, atrioventricular block and intraventricular block.

FIRST DEGREE A-V BLOCK
(Prolonged P–R Interval)

First degree A-V block is a *delay* in conduction through the conducting system. It is reflected by a *prolonged P–R interval*. The P–R interval (sometimes referred to as the P–Q interval) is measured from the *beginning of the P wave* to the *beginning of the QRS complex*, irrespective of whether the QRS complex begins with a Q or R wave (Figs. 162 and 199).

The P–R interval represents (*a*) the time taken for the impulse to

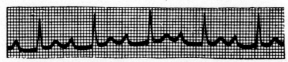

Fig. 162. Electrocardiogram showing first degree A-V block (prolonged P–R interval). The P–R interval, measured from the beginning of the P wave to the beginning of the QRS complex, equals 0.36 sec.

travel from the S-A node to the A-V node (usually 0.03 sec) plus (*b*) the time taken for the impulse to travel through the A-V node, the bundle of His and the bundle branches to the ventricles; this represents by far the greater part of the P–R interval.

In first degree A-V block the P–R interval is prolonged beyond the normal limit of 0.20 sec (beyond 0.18 sec in children). (Figs. 25, 125, 146, 161, 162 and 167.)

Note: In first degree A-V block, *all* the P waves are followed by QRS complexes.

SIGNIFICANCE
First degree A-V block is associated with *coronary artery disease, acute rheumatic carditis* and *digitalis administration.*

SECOND DEGREE A-V BLOCK
('Dropped' Beats)

Second degree A-V block is characterized by an intermittent failure or interruption of A-V conduction. The sinus impulse, after leaving the S-A node and activating the atria to produce the P wave, is blocked within the A-V conducting system. The P wave is therefore *not* followed by a QRS complex and a ventricular beat is 'dropped'. Second degree A-V block thus manifests with regularly occurring P waves, some of which are not followed by QRS complexes.

THE CONDUCTION RATIO
The sequences of second degree A-V block may be expressed in the form of a *conduction ratio*. This is the number of sinus impulses to the number of QRS complexes in any one sequence. A sequence begins with the first conducted sinus beat following a pause created by the 'dropped' beat, ending with, and including the P wave of the ensuing 'dropped' beat. See Figs. 164, 165 and 166 for examples.

Note: Regular 2:1 A-V block will result in a very slow regular ventricular rhythm (Fig. 166). Regular 3:2 A-V block will result in a ventricular bigeminal rhythm (Fig. 165). Variable—irregular—second degree A-V block will result in an irregular ventricular rhythm (Fig. 164).

THE FORMS OF SECOND DEGREE A-V BLOCK

The sinus impulses may be blocked at *regular or irregular intervals,* and the 'dropped' beat may be preceded by *constant P–R intervals* or by a *progressive increase in P–R intervals.* These manifestations result in the following varieties of second degree A-V block.

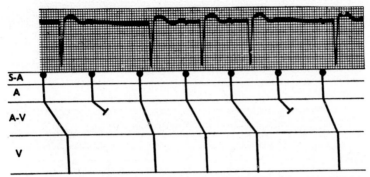

FIG. 163. Electrocardiogram (lead V3) showing second degree A-V block of the Wenckebach type. Note (a) that following a 'dropped' beat, the P–R interval becomes progressively longer until another beat is 'dropped'; (b) the atrial rhythm is regular and all the P waves are present; it is thus the QRS complex that is 'dropped'; (c) the infarction pattern in the QRS complex. From a case of anterior myocardial infarction.

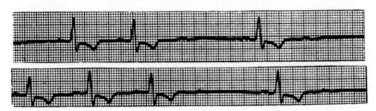

FIG. 164. Electrocardiogram (continuous strip of Standard lead II) showing second degree A-V block with fixed P–R interval. Note (a) beats are 'dropped' irregularly as a result of successive 3:2, 2:1, 4:3 and 2:1 A-V block; (b) the P–R interval is prolonged (0.26 sec) but is the same for all conducted beats; (c) the **P. mitrale.**

I. SECOND DEGREE A-V BLOCK WITH THE WENCKEBACH PHENOMENON

Synonym: Mobitz Type I A-V Block

In this type of second degree A-V block, transmission through the conducting system becomes increasingly difficult until it fails completely and a beat is 'dropped'. The sequence begins with a normal or prolonged P–R interval; and with each successive beat the P–R interval lengthens until a beat is 'dropped'. The pause occasioned by the 'dropped' beat allows the conducting system to recover and the sequence is then repeated (Figs. 163 and 165). The defect or mechanism giving rise to this form of second degree A-V block may be situated in the A-V

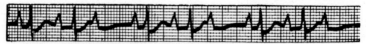

FIG. 165. Electrocardiogram (Standard lead II) showing bigeminal rhythm due to regularly recurring 3:2 A-V block of the Wenckebach type.

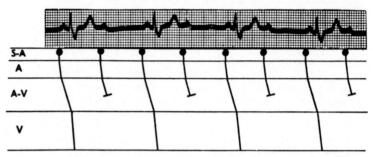

FIG. 166. Electrocardiogram showing 2:1 A-V block. Note (*a*) the sinus rhythm is regular; (*b*) every second P wave is not followed by a QRS complex; (*c*) the consequent slow ventricular rate.

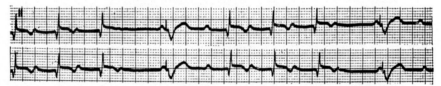

FIG. 167. Electrocardiogram (continuous strip of Standard lead II) showing: 1. *Acute myocardial infarction.* This is reflected by the pathological Q waves, raised, coved S-T segments and inverted T waves. 2. *Normal sinus rhythm.* 3. *First degree A-V block.* The P–R intervals measure 0.36 sec. 4. *Mobitz Type II second degree A-V block.* There is intermittent interruption of conduction. The interruption is preceded by fixed or constant P–R intervals. 5. *Demand pacemaker escape.* The blocked sinus impulse is followed by the escape of an electrical demand pacemaker. Note the pacemaker artifact—the thin vertical line preceding each bizarre QRS complex. The pacemaker beat is dissociated from the near-synchronous P wave.

node itself or within the bundle of His. This form of second degree A-V block may be physiological or pathological.

2. SECOND DEGREE A-V BLOCK WITH FIXED A-V RELATIONSHIP

Synonym: Mobitz Type II A-V Block

In this form of second degree A-V block, the P–R intervals of all the conducted beats are constant, i.e. there is no preceding progressive prolongation of the P–R intervals as occurs in the Wenckebach Phenomenon (Figs. 164 and 167).

The lesion of this form of second degree A-V block is usually situated in the bundle of His, and is always organic or pathological.

THE SIGNIFICANCE OF SECOND DEGREE A-V BLOCK

Second degree A-V block may occur in acute rheumatic carditis, in other forms of acute carditis, e.g. diphtheric carditis, in coronary artery disease, and with digitalis administration.

Second degree A-V block may be associated with fast supraventricular rhythms, e.g. atrial tachycardia and atrial flutter (Figs. 127 and 130). In these conditions, the presence of second degree A-V block is usually physiological; the block only permits every second or third impulse to reach the ventricles, thereby acting as a 'protective' mechanism.

The degree and ratio of the block may fluctuate, e.g. a first degree A-V block may proceed to a second degree A-V block, and a 2:1 ratio may change to a 4:3 ratio.

Atrial tachycardia with a varying 2:1 or 3:2 A-V block is a common manifestation of digitalis intoxication (Fig. 127).

THIRD DEGREE A-V BLOCK: COMPLETE A-V BLOCK

Third degree A-V block is characterized by a complete or permanent interruption of A-V conduction, i.e. all the supraventricular impulses are blocked within the conducting system. The ventricles are then activated by a subsidiary ectopic escape pacemaker situated below the block. The atria are thus activated by one pacemaker—usually the sinus pacemaker, and the ventricles by another. The two rhythms are *asynchronous*, and this results in the following manifestations:

1. *A-V dissociation*
   The *P waves bear no relationship to the QRS complexes.*
2. *A slow ventricular rate*
   The inherent rate of a ventricular pacemaker is slow, and is usually in the range of 30 to 35 beats per minute. A pacemaker situated more proximally, i.e. within the bundle of His, has a slightly faster inherent discharge rate, and is usually in the range of 35 to 45 beats per minute. The inherent discharge of these pacemakers are not under vagal influence. They are thus not usually affected by exercise, emotion, respiration or atropine.

3. *The QRS configuration*

If the subsidiary pacemaker is situated in (*a*) the lower A-V node, i.e. below the block, or (*b*) in the bundle of His, the ectopic impulse activates the ventricles through normal or relatively normal pathways, and the QRS complex is normal in shape (lead V1 in Fig. 168).

If the ectopic pacemaker is situated peripherally in the ventricular musculature, activation of the ventricles is bizarre, and the QRS complex is broad, notched or slurred (Figs. 169, 170 and 171).

At times, two or more subsidiary pacemakers are in competition for the control of the ventricles. Thus, the ventricles may be temporarily under control of one pacemaker resulting in one form of QRS complex, followed by a change of QRS complex when control shifts to the other pacemaker. Stokes-Adams—syncopal—attacks (see below) not infrequently occur with a shift in pacemaker (Fig. 171).

STOKES-ADAMS—SYNCOPAL—ATTACKS

A Stokes-Adams attack is a syncopal attack resulting from ventricular standstill or asystole, and occurs in third degree A-V block when the subsidiary ectopic pacemaker fails to discharge. It is most likely to occur under the following circumstances:

1. During the *transition from incomplete (second degree) to complete (third degree) A-V block* when there may be some delay before a dormant or sluggish pacemaker is aroused and established.

   Note: Complete A-V block that has been stable for a month or longer rarely gives rise to Stokes-Adams attacks.

2. When *two or more ectopic pacemakers are in competition*, a change or shift in pacemaker often heralds a Stokes-Adams attack (Fig. 171).

Syncopal attacks may also be due to paroxysms of ventricular flutter or ventricular fibrillation. These attacks are also sometimes referred to as Stokes-Adams attacks.

'Giant' T wave inversion

When heart rhythm is complicated by ventricular asystole or paroxysmal ventricular flutter or fibrillation—giving rise to syncopal or Stokes-Adams attacks, the electrocardiogram frequently manifests with *very large, broad, bizarre and inverted T waves* (Fig. 168). The phenomenon is usually best seen in leads V2 to V4, and is partly an expression of marked prolongation of the Q–T interval: the Q–Tc may be increased to 180 per cent. The manifestation has been termed 'Giant T wave inversion' (Jacobson & Schrire, 1966[2]), and is virtually pathognomonic of a recent syncopal attack.

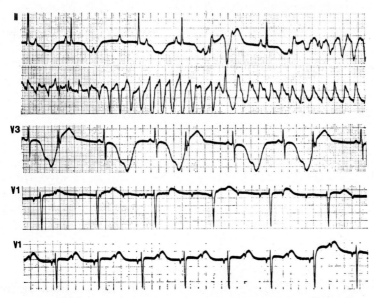

FIG. 168. Electrocardiograms showing: 1. High-grade A-V block. This is evident in the top strip. The second, fourth and seventh QRS complexes are preceded by P–R intervals of 0.14 sec and represent conducted sinus beats. The third and fourth sinus P waves are not conducted and are followed by A-V nodal escape beats. 2. Ventricular flutter. This is represented by the bizarre QRS complexes in Standard lead II which are recorded at a rate of 214 beats per minute. This patient experienced syncopal attacks which were due to the ventricular flutter. 3. 'Giant' T wave inversion and prolonged Q-Tc. This is best seen in lead V3. The manifestation is virtually pathognomonic of preceding episodes of unconsciousness. 3. Complete A-V block. This is evident in lead V1 (upper strip) and followed the administration of intravenous magnesium sulphate. 4. 2:1 A-V block. This occurred two hours later, and is depicted in lead V1 (lower strip).

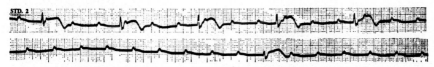

FIG. 169. Electrocardiogram (Standard lead II) showing: 1. *Complete A-V block.* The P waves are unrelated—completely dissociated—from the bizarre QRS complexes of the idioventricular rhythm. The idioventricular rate is 30 beats per minute. 2. *A period of ventricular asystole* (which resulted in a Stokes-Adams attack). The fifth ventricular beat is followed by a period of asystole which is interrupted by a single ventricular beat.

THE CAUSES OF COMPLETE A-V BLOCK

1. IDIOPATHIC SCLERO-DEGENERATIVE DISEASE: 'LENEGRE'S' DISEASE

Many cases of chronic complete A-V block are due to a sclero-degenerative process limited to the conducting system. The cause is unknown. Coronary artery disease does not play a significant role in its pathogenesis. Lenegre (1958)[3] was the first to describe it.

2. CORONARY ARTERY DISEASE

Coronary artery disease, particularly acute myocardial infarction, may cause complete A-V block. The association with acute myocardial infarction usually carries a very adverse prognosis. Indeed, the occurrence of any form of A-V block as a complication of acute myocardial infarction worsens the prognosis. The higher the degree of block, the worse the prognosis (Cohen and associates, 1958[1]).

3. FIBROCALCAREOUS ENCROACHMENT: 'LEV'S' DISEASE

Complete A-V block may result from the extension of a fibrocalcareous process which may involve the aortic valve (aortic stenosis), the pars membranacea, the mitral annulus, and the summit of the interventricular septum. Encroachment of the disease process upon the neighbouring conducting system may cause complete A-V block. The condition usually occurs in elderly people and has received emphasis by Lev (1964).[4]

4. INTRACARDIAC SURGERY

Surgery in the vicinity of the conducting system may cause complete A-V block either by direct severance of the conducting system, or as a result of oedema and pressure upon the conducting system.

5. DIGITALIS INTOXICATION

Digitalis intoxication may rarely cause complete A-V block. When this occurs, there is usually a concomitant underlying pathology such as degenerative or coronary artery disease. In other words, digitalis intoxication rarely causes third degree A-V block unless there is some associated disease; whereas it readily causes first or second degree A-V block.

6. TUMOURS, PARASITIC INFESTATIONS, PYOGENIC AND GRANULOMATOUS INFECTIONS

These diseases may involve the conducting system and cause complete A-V block. They are, however, very rare causes of complete A-V block and may be regarded as clinical curiosities.

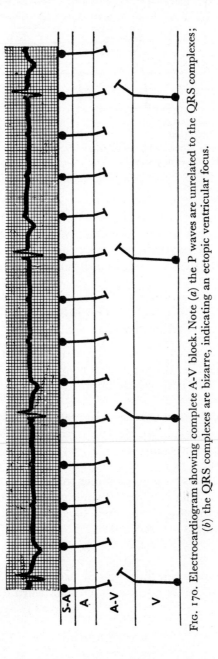

FIG. 170. Electrocardiogram showing complete A-V block. Note (*a*) the P waves are unrelated to the QRS complexes; (*b*) the QRS complexes are bizarre, indicating an ectopic ventricular focus.

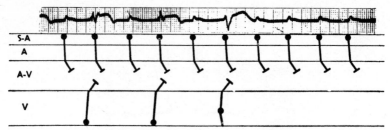

Fig. 171. Electrocardiogram showing complete A-V block. Note (*a*) the P waves are unrelated to the QRS complexes; (*b*) the QRS complexes are bizarre indicating an ectopic ventricular origin; (*c*) the third QRS complex differs from the other two indicating a change in ventricular focus; this change precipitates cardiac, or ventricular, standstill—a Stokes-Adams attack.

7. CONGENITAL HEART DISEASE

Complete A-V block is not infrequently associated with congenital heart disease such as corrected transposition of the great vessels, ventricular septal defect and ostium primum type of atrial septal defect.

8. CONGENITAL A-V BLOCK

Complete A-V block may occur as an isolated congenital anomaly. It has the following electrocardiographic features:

A. The block is nearly always within the A-V node and the sub-sidiary pacemaker is situated just below the block within the lower part of the A-V node or the bundle of His. *The QRS complexes are therefore normal.*

B. The idionodal rate is usually in the rate-range of 55 to 65 beats per minute, i.e. in a slightly higher rate-range than that usually associated with acquired complete A-V block.

C. The ventricular rate tends to fluctuate slightly with emotion and exercise, i.e. it appears to be under some autonomic influence and is therefore less stable than the rhythm usually associated with the acquired forms of complete A-V block.

D. Syncopal attacks are very rare.

Note: Acute rheumatic carditis may be associated with first or second degree A-V block, but is not associated with third degree or complete A-V block.

REFERENCES

1   COHEN D. B., DOCTOR L. & PICK A. (1958) The significance of atrioventricular block complicating acute myocardial infarction. *Amer. Heart J.* **55,** 215.

2 JACOBSON D. & SCHRIVE V. (1966) Giant T-wave inversion. *Brit. Heart J.* **28,** 768.

3 LENEGRE J. (1958) *Contribution a l'Etude des Blocs de Branche.* Paris: J. B. Ballière et Fils.

4 LEV M. (1964) Anatomic basis of atrioventricular block. *Amer. J. Med.* **37,** 742.

CHAPTER 18

Phasic Aberrant Ventricular Conduction

An isolated, bizarre QRS complex is not necessarily the result of an ectopic ventricular discharge but may be due to *temporary* abnormal intraventricular conduction (bundle branch block). This isolated form of bundle branch block occurs during rhythm that otherwise shows normal intraventricular conduction. Lewis (1912)[1] termed this condition **aberrant ventricular conduction** and defined it as the abnormal intraventricular conduction of a supraventricular impulse. Strict interpretation of this definition, however, makes it applicable to both the temporary *and* permanent forms of abnormal intraventricular conduction. To define these conditions more accurately, the term **phasic** aberrant ventricular conduction was introduced to distinguish the temporary form from the **non-phasic** or permanent form of aberrant ventricular conduction (Schamroth & Chesler, 1963[8]).

Aberrant ventricular conduction results in a bizarre QRS complex resembling left or right bundle branch block. In phasic aberrant ventricular conduction these bizarre QRS complexes occur during rhythms which otherwise show normal intraventricular conduction. Thus, phasic aberrant ventricular conduction may mimic the bizarre complexes found in ventricular ectopic rhythms, e.g. paroxysmal—extrasystolic—ventricular tachycardia. The recognition of phasic aberrant ventricular conduction is thus of major clinical import, since the differentiation of supraventricular from ventricular rhythms affects both prognosis and treatment.

MECHANISM

Phasic aberrant ventricular conduction may complicate any supraventricular rhythm, viz. sinus rhythm, A-V nodal rhythm, atrial and A-V nodal extrasystoles, paroxysmal atrial and A-V nodal tachycardias, atrial flutter and atrial fibrillation. The disturbance is dependent upon:

1. **Unequal refractory periods of the bundle branches.**
2. **Early impulse formation.**
3. **The length of the preceding R–R interval.**

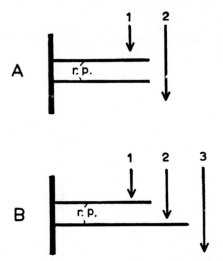

FIG. 172. Diagram illustrating the refractory periods (r.p.) of the bundle branches and their effect on subsequent impulse formation. (A) with equal refractory periods of the bundle branches; (B) with unequal refractory periods of the bundle branches.

When the refractory periods of the bundle branches are equal (Fig. 172A), an impulse which occurs relatively late (at position 2) will find both bundle branches fully recovered and will be conducted with normal intraventricular conduction. An impulse which occurs very early (at position 1) will find both bundles refractory and will be blocked, and there will be no intraventricular conduction.

When the refractory periods of the bundle branches are unequal (Fig. 172B), an impulse which occurs relatively late (at position 3) will be conducted with normal intraventricular conduction. An impulse falling very early—at position 1—will be blocked; an impulse falling at position 2, i.e. between positions 1 and 3, will find one bundle branch recovered and the other refractory—it will thus be conducted down one bundle branch only, resulting in the bizarre QRS pattern of bundle branch block. It is usually the left bundle branch that recovers first and thus phasic aberrant ventricular conduction commonly, though not invariably, results in a right bundle branch block pattern. Hence it will be seen that **unequal refractory periods are essential to the occurrence of phasic aberrant ventricular conduction**, and that the phenomenon is **favoured by early or premature impulses**—the earlier the impulse, within limits, the more likely it is to find one of the bundle branches refractory.

These phenomena are illustrated in Figs. 173, 174, 175, 177, 178, 179, 180 and 184. Fig. 173 shows atrial extrasystoles: very early extrasystoles

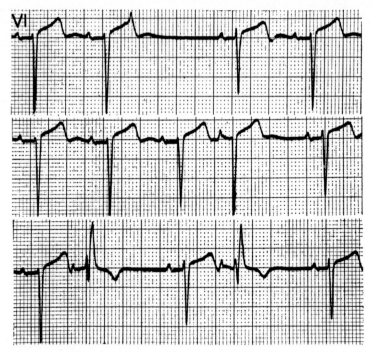

FIG. 173. Electrocardiogram (non-continuous strips of lead V1) illustrating:

A. *Top strip.* A blocked—non-conducted—atrial extrasystole. The premature bizarre P wave is superimposed upon the T wave of the second sinus beat.

B. *Middle strip.* A normally conducted atrial extrasystole. The fourth P wave is premature and bizarre. It is, however, *relatively* late (compare with top strip) and is therefore conducted normally.

C. *Bottom strip.* Atrial extrasystoles conducted with phasic aberrant. ventricular conduction. The second and fourth P waves are premature, bizarre, and followed by QRS complexes showing the right bundle branch block pattern of phasic aberrant ventricular conduction. Note the timing of these extrasystoles is in between the extrasystoles of the top and middle strips.

are blocked; late extrasystoles are conducted with normal intraventricular conduction, extrasystoles intermediate in timing are conducted with aberration. Fig. 174 is an example of intermittent bundle branch block dependent upon critical rate (Vesell, 1941[11]; Shearn & Rytand, 1953[9]). With a relatively slow heart rate, the sinus impulses find both bundle branches fully recovered and are normally conducted (mechanism illustrated by position 3 in Diagram B of Fig. 172). With an increase in heart rate, the sinus impulses find the left bundle branch refractory and the right bundle branch responsive; and are therefore conducted with

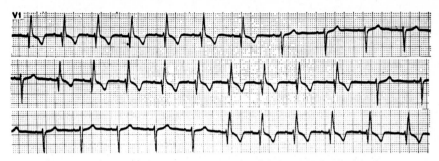

FIG. 174. Electrocardiogram (continuous strip of lead V1) showing sinus rhythm with bundle branch block dependent upon critical rate. There is slight sinus arrhythmia. The shorter cycles are associated with right bundle branch block conduction—a manifestation of phasic aberrant ventricular conduction. The longer cycles are associated with normal intraventricular conduction.

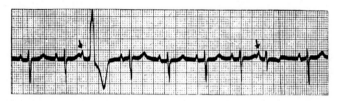

FIG. 175. Electrocardiogram showing atrial extrasystoles (marked with arrows) conducted with different degrees of aberration.

the right bundle branch block pattern of phasic aberrant ventricular conduction (mechanism illustrated by position 2 in Diagram B of Fig. 172).

The significance of the preceding R–R interval

The duration of the refractory period is directly proportional to the length of the preceding R–R interval (Fig. 176). With a long preceding R–R interval the subsequent refractory period will be relatively long (illustrated in Diagram A II of Fig. 176); with a shorter preceding R–R interval the subsequent refractory period will be relatively shorter (illustrated in Diagram A I of Fig. 176). In other words, the refractory period shortens with tachycardia and lengthens with bradycardia (Trendelenburg, 1903[10]; Mines, 1913[6]; Lewis, Drury & Bulger, 1921[2]). The same principle applies in the presence of unequal refractory periods of the bundle branches. When the preceding R–R interval is relatively short, the subsequent refractory periods of the bundle branches will be relatively short (illustrated in Diagram B I of Fig. 176). When this occurs, an early beat—X—will find both bundle branches recovered

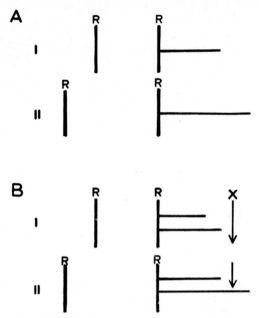

FIG. 176. Diagram illustrating the effect of long and short R–R intervals on the ensuing refractory period(s).

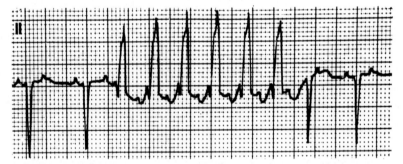

FIG. 177. The electrocardiogram (Standard lead II) begins with a conducted sinus impulse. This is followed by a blocked atrial extrasystole. The P′ wave of the atrial extrasystole is superimposed upon the T wave of the sinus beat. The coupling interval of the atrial extrasystole (P–P′ interval) measures 0.25 sec. The extrasystolic impulse is very premature and therefore encounters refractory A-V nodal tissue. The extrasystole is followed by another conducted sinus beat which in turn is followed by a further atrial extrasystole. This atrial extrasystole, however, occurs slightly later: the coupling interval (P–P′ interval) measures 0.29 sec. This impulse finds the A-V node and the left bundle branch responsive, and is consequently conducted to the ventricles with phasic aberrant ventricular conduction—a right bundle branch block pattern. This is followed by a paroxysm of successive atrial extrasystoles —an extrasystolic atrial tachycardia—which is conducted with the same form of aberration. *Note*: Every bizarre QRS complex is related to a preceding P′ wave.

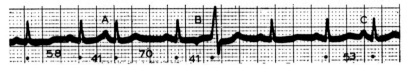

FIG. 178. Electrocardiogram showing three atrial extrasystoles (labelled A, B and C). Extrasystole C occurs relatively late and is thus normally conducted. Extrasystoles A and B result in QRS complexes which occur at the same interval (0.41 sec) from the preceding sinus beat; A is normally conducted as it is preceded by a relatively short R–R interval (0.58 sec); B is conducted with aberration as it is preceded by a relatively long R–R interval (0.70 sec). All time intervals are indicated in hundredths of a second.

STD. 2

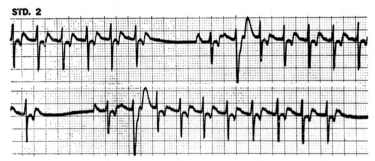

FIG. 179. Electrocardiogram (continuous strip of Standard lead II) showing paroxysms of superventricular tachycardia (a form of reciprocal rhythm with retrograde atrial activation). Note that only the second QRS complex of each paroxysm is conducted with aberration; this is because it is only the second atrial impulse of each paroxysm that is preceded by a long R–R interval.

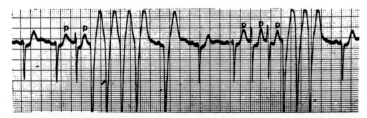

FIG. 180. Electrocardiogram showing paroxysms of atrial tachycardia conducted with aberration. The P waves (labelled) are seen before the bizarre QRS complexes at the beginning of each paroxysm; they are superimposed on the preceding T waves. Note the increasing abnormality of the QRS complexes as the rate speeds up. P waves cannot be distinguished during the 'full-blown' established tachycardia and the paroxysm then resembles ventricular tachycardia.

and will be conducted normally. With a relatively long preceding R–R interval the subsequent refractory periods of the bundle branches will be relatively long (illustrated in Diagram B II of Fig. 176) and an early impulse—X—(of the same prematurity as illustrated in Diagram B I)—will now find one bundle branch refractory and is therefore conducted with ventricular aberration. **Phasic aberrant ventricular conduction is thus favoured by a long preceding R–R interval.** This is illustrated in Fig. 178. The tracing shows three atrial extrasystoles—A, B and C. Extrasystoles A and B result in identical R–R intervals (0.41 sec), yet extrasystole A is conducted normally whereas extrasystole B is conducted with ventricular aberration. This is because B is preceded by a long R–R interval (0.70 sec), whereas extrasystole A is preceded by a short R–R interval (0.58 sec).

This principle is also illustrated in Fig. 179 where *only the second beat* of a run of paroxysmal supraventricular tachycardia shows aberrant ventricular conduction—a pattern that may almost be regarded as a hallmark of phasic aberrant ventricular conduction. This occurs because only the second beat of the paroxysm is preceded by a long R–R interval, whereas the subsequent beats of the tachycardia are preceded by short R–R intervals. If, however, the second and subsequent beats occur *very* early, then all the beats except the first may be conducted with ventricular aberration (Fig. 180). The same principle may be evident in cases of atrial flutter with alternating 4:1 and 2:1 A-V block (see page 192 and Figs. 184 and 185).

THE DIFFERENTIATION OF ECTOPIC VENTRICULAR RHYTHMS FROM SUPRA-VENTRICULAR RHYTHMS WITH PHASIC ABERRANT VENTRICULAR CONDUCTION

The differentiation of ectopic ventricular rhythms from supraventricular rhythms conducted with phasic aberrant ventricular conduction is based primarily on two electrocardiographic principles:

1. The P:QRS relationship.
2. The morphology of the QRS complex.

1. *The P: QRS relationship*

Among the more important aspects in the diagnosis of the arrhythmias, is the identification of the P waves and their relationship to the QRS complexes. For the diagnosis of supraventricular tachycardia with phasic aberrant ventricular conduction, it must be shown that the bizarre QRS complexes are **related to preceding atrial deflections**. In ectopic ventricular tachycardia, the P waves are dissociated from the QRS complexes, or, in the case of retrograde A-V

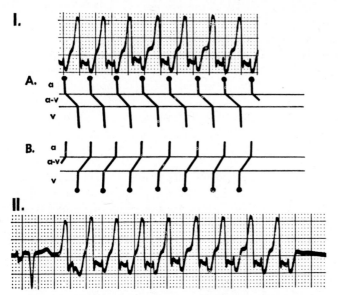

FIG. 181. Electrocardiogram (lead V1). Illustration I shows a tachycardia which is reflected by the bizarre QRS complexes. Each QRS complex is related to a bizarre P' wave. However, it is impossible to tell whether this represents extrasystolic atrial tachycardia with phasic aberrant ventricular conduction (as illustrated in Diagram A) or extrasystolic ventricular tachycardia with retrograde A-V conduction (as illustrated in Diagram B). Definitive diagnosis is possible when the beginning of the tachycardia is observed (illustration II). The first bizarre QRS complex is now seen to be followed by a P' wave, i.e. it is not related to a preceding P' wave. This, as well as the form of the QRS complex, establishes the ventricular origin of the tachycardia (as illustrated in Diagram I B).

conduction of the ventricular impulses, the bizarre QRS complexes are **related to ensuing P' deflections**. This relationship may be obscured with very fast rhythms when the P waves are hidden within the QRS complexes and the S-T segments. And even if the P waves can be identified, it may be impossible to establish the true P:QRS relationship. For example, in some cases of paroxysmal tachycardia it may not be possible to tell whether the P':QRS relationship represents (a) an ectopic atrial impulse with aberrant anterograde conduction to the ventricles, or (b) a ventricular impulse with retrograde conduction to the atria. This is illustrated in Fig. 181. Electrocardiogram 1 reveals a close relationship between the P' deflections and the bizarre QRS complexes: every QRS complex is related to a P' deflection. This relationship, however, could represent (i) a ventricular tachycardia with retrograde conduction to the atria; every QRS complex would then be related to the ensuing P' deflection (as illustrated in Diagram B of Fig. 181), or (ii) an ectopic atrial tachycardia with aberrant anterograde conduction to the ventricles; every QRS complex would then be related to the preceding P' deflection (as illustrated in Diagram A of Fig. 181). The situation becomes clarified when the beginning of the paroxysm is observed (as shown in Diagram II of Fig. 181). It is now evident that the first abnormal QRS complex of the paroxysm is *followed* by the P' deflection and the rhythm is therefore a ventricular tachycardia with retrograde conduction to the atria.

The ventricular origin of the tachycardia is also suggested by the fact that the morphology of the QRS complexes is diphasic (almost monophasic) but not triphasic, and does not resemble either classic right or left bundle branch block (see below).

Note that A-V dissociation between P waves and bizarre QRS complexes does not necessarily connote ectopic ventricular origin since the bizarre QRS complexes may be the expression of an A-V nodal tachycardia with aberrant ventricular conduction. In such a circumstance the differentiation must be based on the morphology of the QRS complex (see below).

2. *The Morphology of the QRS complex*

The P:QRS relationship may, at times, be difficult if not impossible to establish. It may, for example, be difficult to establish whether the P waves are related to ensuing or preceding QRS complexes (Fig. 181). And, with very rapid tachyarrhythmias the P waves may be difficult to identify because they are obscured by the QRS complexes (Fig. 180). Furthermore, in cases of atrial fibrillation, it is clearly impossible to establish a P:QRS relationship. Under these circumstances reliance must be placed on the morphology of the QRS complex which although not absolutely pathognomonic of either aberration or ventricular ectopy, nevertheless provides strong diagnostic indication of one or the other condition. These morphological characteristics are considered below.

The significance of the QRS configuration

The features are best observed in lead V1 or lead MCL1 (Marriott and Fogg, 1970[5]; Fig. 182). This lead is formed by placing the positive pole of a bipolar monitoring lead on the lead V1 position, and the negative pole on the left shoulder just under the outer end of the clavicle (Fig. 182).

In contrast to the usual monitoring bipolar lead placed on either side of the sternum, the MCL1 lead has the advantage that it does not inter-

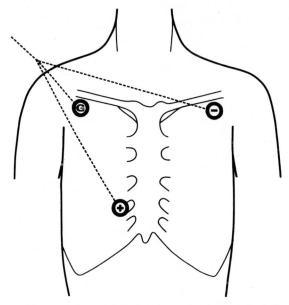

FIG. 182. Diagram illustrating the electrode placement of the MCL1 lead.[5]

fere unduly with auscultation and other physical examination of the heart, it does not interfere with the administration of precordial electric shock, and it is less cumbersome for nursing the patient.

The ensuing section is based mainly on the elegant studies of Marriott and his associates.[3, 4, 5, 7]

The significance of the initial vector. Most examples of phasic aberrant ventricular conduction reflect a right bundle branch block pattern. Right bundle branch block does not alter the initial vector of the QRS deflection (see Chapter 3 and Fig. 65). Hence the initial vectors of the QRS complex will tend to the same during both normal intraventricular conduction and phasic aberrant ventricular conduction (Figs. 173, 174 and 184). In ventricular ectopy, however, the initial vectors are usually markedly different (Fig. 181).

The significance of the triphasic configuration.[7] The QRS complex of right bundle branch block characteristically has a triphasic configuration, an rsR variant in lead V1 and a qRS variant in lead V6 (Diagram B of Fig. 65). The initial vectors (the rS deflection in right ventricular leads, and the qR deflection in left ventricular leads) are essentially unchanged. The right bundle branch merely results in the addition of a terminal deflection, an anterior and rightward directed

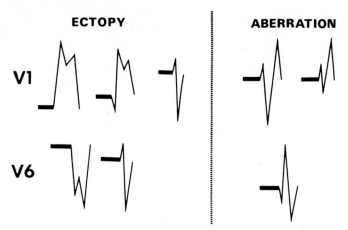

FIG. 183. Diagrams illustrating the QRS manifestations of ventricular ectopy and ventricular aberration.

vector. Hence, phasic aberrant ventricular conduction is usually associated with a triphasic configuration in lead V1. Similarly, a qRs complex in lead V6 is also an expression of right bundle branch block, and favours phasic aberrant ventricular conduction (Diagram B of Fig. 65 and Fig. 183). Ventricular ectopy, however, tends to have a monophasic or diphasic configuration in leads V1 or V6, a wide and bizarre dominantly upward or dominantly negative deflection with a notched apex or nadir (Fig. 183). Furthermore, the QRS complex of ventricular ectopy is completely bizarre, and does not resemble the classic forms of either right or left bundle branch block (Figs. 149 and 181).

The significance of the relative amplitude of the R and R′ deflections: the significance of the QRS 'Rabbit Ears'. When lead V1 or lead MCL1 reflects a bizarre, dominantly upright QRS complex with a notched apex, and the initial deflection of the QRS complex, the R wave, is taller than the second deflection of the QRS complex, the R′ wave, ventricular ectopy is the most likely diagnosis (Fig. 183). The notched upright QRS complex has been likened to a pair of rabbit ears,[3, 4] and when the first or left rabbit ear (viewing the rabbit from behind) of the QRS configuration is taller than the second rabbit ear, ventricular ectopy is the likely diagnosis. This may occasionally be preceded by a small initial q wave (Fig. 183).

The significance of the concordant pattern. If the electrocardiogram presents with a series of bizarre QRS complexes which are dominantly positive in *all* the precordial leads, ventricular ectopy is the most likely diagnosis (Fig. 149). The only other condition with a similar presentation is the Type A Wolff-Parkinson-White syndrome with atrial fibrillation, in which case the rhythm will be markedly irregular.

The significance of an rS or RS complex in lead V1. An rS or RS complex in lead V1 with a rather broad initial r or R wave usually indicates right ventricular ectopy (Fig. 183).

The significance of an rS complex in leads V5 and V6. An rS complex in leads V5 and V6 is usually due to ventricular ectopy (Fig. 183). It may also be due to:

(*a*) Right bundle branch block with left anterior hemiblock.
(*b*) Marked right ventricular dominance.
(*c*) Mirror-image dextrocardia.

Thus, when the features of the latter three conditions can be excluded (and this does not usually present any great difficulty), the presence of an rS complex in leads V5 and V6 connotes ventricular ectopy.

The significance of the mean frontal plane QRS axis. Phasic aberrant ventricular conduction is usually associated with a normal or near normal frontal plane QRS axis, for example, in the range of 0° to +90° or 100°, whereas ventricular ectopy is commonly associated with a bizarre QRS axis, for example −150° (Fig. 149).

The significance of a QS complex in lead V6. A QS complex— a wide, notched and entirely negative complex—in lead V6 usually connotes ventricular ectopy (Fig. 183).

The significance of ventricular fusion complexes. One of the best signs of ectopic ventricular origin is the presence of a ventricular fusion complex. This complex results from fortuitous concomitant activation of the ventricles by a supraventricular impulse and a ventricular impulse. The resulting QRS complex thus has a configuration that is in between that of the pure ectopic beat and the pure conducted supraventricular beat (see Chapter 13, page 155). Examples of all three complexes must be present in the same tracing before the diagnosis can be established.

The significance of the compensatory pause. When phasic aberrant ventricular conduction complicates atrial fibrillation, the bizarre QRS complex of the aberration is not usually nor necessarily followed by a compensatory pause, or an attempt at a compensatory pause. When, however, a ventricular extrasystole, for example, complicates atrial fibrillation, the bizarre QRS complex is usually followed by a long or relatively long pause. This is due to concealed retrograde conduction of the extrasystolic impulse into the A-V node, thereby rendering it refractory to the immediately ensuing fibrillation impulses.

ATRIAL FLUTTER WITH ABERRANT VENTRICULAR CONDUCTION SIMULATING EXTRASYSTOLIC VENTRICULAR BIGEMINY

Phasic aberrant ventricular conduction is particularly prone to occur during atrial flutter, when relatively early conducted beats may be conducted with aberration, and may consequently mimic extrasystolic ventricular rhythm.

MECHANISM

The manifestation of aberrant ventricular conduction during atrial flutter is basically due to the presence of alternating 4:1 and 2:1 atrioventricular (A-V) block. This will result in a form of ventricular bigeminal rhythm, since the 2:1 A-V block results in two beats which are inscribed in relatively quick succession, whereas the 4:1 A-V block results in a relatively long pause. Furthermore, the conducted impulse

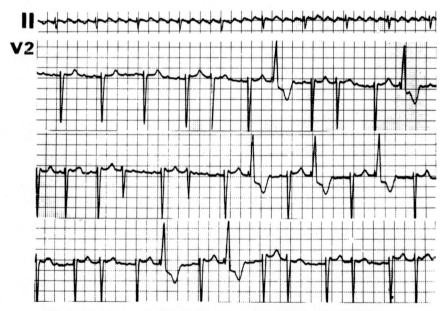

FIG. 184. Electrocardiogram showing atrial flutter with variable 4:1 and 2:1 A-V block. The impulses are conducted with normal intraventricular conduction and with aberration (see text).

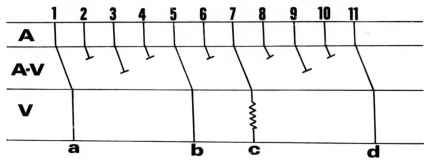

FIG. 185. Diagram illustrating atrial flutter with alternating 4:1 and 2:1 A-V block. The conducted impulse beginning a 4:1 conduction sequence is conducted with aberration.

terminating the 2:1 A-V block is premature and is, therefore, likely to be conducted with aberration. In addition, it is preceded by a long pause—the period of 4:1 A-V block. And since a long pause results in an ensuing prolongation of refractoriness, this too will favour the ensuing aberration.

The mechanism and principle are diagrammatically illustrated in Fig. 185. Impulses 1 to 11 represent flutter impulses. The conducted impulses—1, 5, 7, and 11—are also labelled a, b, c, and d. Beat c terminates the 2:1 episode of A-V block and is, therefore, relatively premature. It is consequently conducted with aberration. Furthermore, it is preceded by a relatively long ventricular cycle—the preceding period of 4:1 A-V conduction. This favours an ensuing prolongation of refractoriness. The second beat of the bigeminal couplet is consequently conducted with aberration and mimics extrasystolic ventricular bigeminy. This manifestation is illustrated in Fig. 184.

The electrocardiogram (a strip of Standard lead II, and a continuous strip of lead V2) was recorded from a 40-year-old man with congestive cardiac failure due to a congestive cardiomyopathy. He was not on digitalis therapy.

Standard lead II shows atrial flutter with 4:1 A-V block. Lead V2 shows the following:

1. Periods of uncomplicated 4:1 A-V block—the first four beats of the tracing.
2. A period of 4:1 A-V block alternating with 2:1 A-V block, and associated with normal intraventricular conduction—the last six beats of the bottom strip.
3. The second half of the middle strip reflects three bizarre QRS complexes alternating with normal QRS complexes. This simulates extrasystolic ventricular bigeminy. Analysis, however, reveals that these

are most likely to be aberrantly conducted flutter impulses which terminate cycles of 2:1 A-V conduction. This is evident from the following characteristics of the aberration:

(a) The initial QRS vector of the abnormal QRS complex is the same as that of the normally conducted QRS complex.
(b) The QRS complex has a triphasic configuration.[7]
(c) Beats 4 and 6 of the middle strip show lesser degrees of aberration.
(d) The pause following the bizarre beat is identical to the pause created by the 4:1 A-V conduction with normal intraventricular conduction.

Comment

The accurate differentiation of phasic aberrant ventricular conduction from ventricular ectopic conduction is of particular importance in the context of atrial flutter, since the diagnosis of aberration would be an indication to begin or increase the digitalis therapy, whereas the diagnosis of extrasystolic ventricular bigeminy would be an indication to stop digitalis therapy, or to proceed with caution.

REFERENCES

1 LEWIS T. (1912) Observations upon disorders of the heart's action. *Heart* **3**, 279.
2 LEWIS T., DRURY A. N. & BULGER (1921) Observations upon flutter and fibrillation. Part VI. *Heart* **8**, 83.
3 MARRIOTT H. J. L. (1972) *Practical Electrocardiography*, 4th Edition. Baltimore: Williams and Wilkins Co.
4 MARRIOTT H. J. L. (1972) *Workshop in Electrocardiography*. Oldmar, Florida: Tampa Tracings.
5 MARRIOTT H. J. L. & FOGG E. (1970) Constant monitoring for cardiac dysrrhythmias and blocks. *Mod. Conc. Cardiovasc. Dis.* **39**, 103.
6 MINES G. R. (1913) On dynamic equilibrium in the heart. *J. Physiol.* (*Lond.*) **46**, 349.
7 SANDLER A. & MARRIOTT H. J. L. (1965) The differential morphology of anomalous ventricular complexes of right bundle branch block-type in Lead V_1. Ventricular ectopic versus aberration. *Circulation* **31**, 551.
8 SCHAMROTH L. & CHESLER E. (1963) Phasic aberrant ventricular conduction. *Brit. Heart J.* **25**, 219.
9 SHEARN M. A. & RYTAND D. A. (1953) Intermittent bundle branch block: observations with special reference to the critical heart rate. *Arch. intern. Med.* **91**, 440.
10 TRENDELENBURG W. (1903) Ueber den Wegfall der Compensatorischen Ruhe am spontan Schlagenden/Froschherzen. *Arch. Anat. Physiol.* (*Lps.*) *Physiol. Abt.* 311.
11 VESELL H. (1941) Critical rate in ventricular conduction: unstable bundle branch block. *Amer. J. med. Sci.* **202**, 198.

CHAPTER 19

The Wolff-Parkinson-White Syndrome

The Wolff-Parkinson-White (W-P-W) syndrome (1930)[3] is an electro-cardiographic syndrome resulting from concomitant normal and anomalous conduction of the atrial impulse to the ventricles. It has the following characteristics (Figs. 186, 188, 191, 192 and 193).

1. **A shortened P–R interval.**
2. **A widened QRS complex.**
3. A slurred and thickened proximal limb of the QRS complex—designated the **delta wave**.

The P–R interval is shortened by as much as the QRS complex is widened, as though the proximal limb of the QRS complex has been 'pulled towards' the P wave (Fig. 186).

MECHANISM

The abnormality is due to the presence of an *anomalous pathway*—an additional A-V pathway or by-pass—probably congenital in origin,

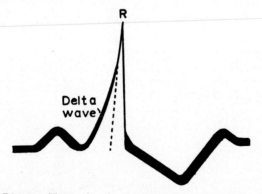

FIG. 186. Diagram illustrating the electrocardiographic deflections of the W-P-W syndrome. Note (*a*) the short P–R interval; (*b*) the slurred upstroke of the QRS complex—the delta wave; (*c*) the widened QRS complex. The dotted line indicates the normal position of the proximal limb of the QRS complex.

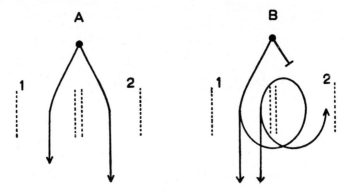

FIG. 187. Diagrams illustrating the conduction mechanisms in the W-P-W syndrome. (1) Normal pathway, i.e. the A-V node. (2) Anomalous pathway. (A) illustrates the conduction mechanism that inscribes the typical W-P-W pattern, i.e. the atrial impulse is conducted through both pathways concomitantly but at a faster rate through the anomalous pathway. (B) illustrates conduction during paroxysmal tachycardia, viz. anterogradely through the normal pathway and retrogradely through the anomalous pathway.

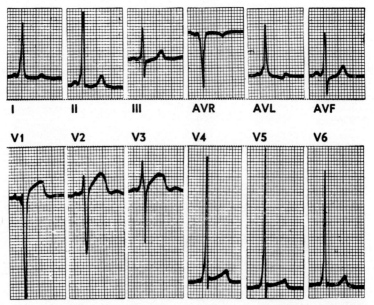

FIG. 188. Electrocardiogram showing the W-P-W syndrome. Note the short P–R interval, delta wave, and widened QRS complex—well seen in most leads.

between the atria and ventricles (Figs. 187, 189 and 190). The pathway may be situated anywhere along the A-V ring.

The atrial impulse travels down *both* the normal and anomalous pathways concomitantly (Figs. 187A and 190A) but is conducted at a faster rate down the anomalous pathway. It thus reaches the ventricles earlier than the normally conducted impulse and results in the early inscription of the QRS complex—hence the shortened P–R interval. Once this impulse reaches the ventricles, however, further onward or caudal transmission is not through specialized conducting tissue but through ordinary myocardium which is a poor conducting medium. Further conduction is therefore slower than normal, producing the bizarre, slurred, delta wave.

Conduction through the A-V node proceeds normally but at a slower rate than through the anomalous pathway. Once it reaches the ventricles, however, further transmission is through normal, quick conducting specialized tissue, viz. the bundle branches and Purkinje network. Consequently, the impulse conducted through the A-V node eventually 'overtakes' the impulse conducted through the anomalous pathway and records the rest of the QRS complex which is therefore normal. Thus the typical complex of the W-P-W syndrome is a form of **fusion complex**: the initial part—the delta wave—is recorded by the impulse conducted through the anomalous pathway; and the normal part of the QRS complex is recorded by the impulse conducted through the A-V node.

THE TYPE A AND TYPE B W-P-W SYNDROME

The W-P-W syndrome may be classified into two types, based on the direction of the dominant QRS deflection in the right precordial leads: leads V1 and V2 (Rosenbaum and associates, 1945[1]).

THE TYPE A W-P-W SYNDROME

The Type A W-P-W syndrome is characterized by a dominantly upright QRS deflection in the right precordial leads, resulting in tall R waves in leads V1 and V2 (Fig. 191).

The by-pass in the Type A W-P-W syndrome is usually situated on the left, i.e. the pre-excitation area is usually the left ventricle.

THE TYPE B W-P-W SYNDROME

The Type B W-P-W syndrome is characterized by a dominantly negative QRS deflection in the right precordial leads (Fig. 188).

When the Type B W-P-W syndrome is associated with cyanotic congenital heart disease, it is said to be pathognomonic of Ebstein's Anomaly (Sodi-Pallares & Calder, 1956[2]).

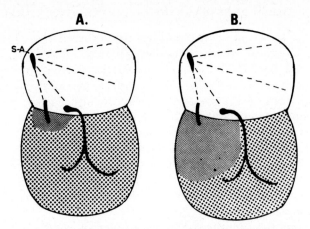

FIG. 189. Diagrams illustrating the typical conduction of the W-P-W syndrome. The darker shading reflects the pre-excitation area: the contribution to ventricular activation by the impulse conducted through the by-pass. Pre-excitation is greater in Diagram B than in Diagram A.

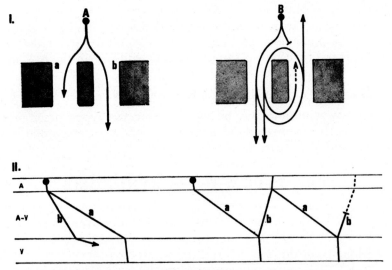

FIG. 190. Diagrams illustrating the conduction mechanisms of the W-P-W syndrome. (a) represents conduction through the normal pathway. (b) represents conduction through the anomalous pathway.

Diagram A illustrates the conduction mechanism responsible for the typical W-P-W pattern, i.e. the sinus impulse is conducted through both pathways concomitantly but at a faster rate through the anomalous pathway. Diagram B illustrates the conduction mechanism responsible for the reciprocating—paroxysmal—tachycardia, i.e. antero-grade conduction through the normal pathway and retrograde conduction through the anomalous pathway.

The by-pass in the Type B W-P-W syndrome is usually situated on the right, i.e. the pre-excitation area is usually in the right ventricle.

THE SIGNIFICANCE OF THE W-P-W SYNDROME

The W-P-W syndrome has two important implications:

1. Individuals with the W-P-W syndrome are prone to attacks of **supraventricular tachyarrhythmias**:

   A. Reciprocating tachycardia.
   B. Paroxysmal atrial flutter or paroxysmal atrial fibrillation.

2. The W-P-W syndrome may mimic other electrocardiographic manifestations and lead to erroneous diagnosis.

1. THE SUPRAVENTRICULAR TACHYARRHYTHMIAS
A. *Reciprocating tachycardia*
Anterograde conduction through the anomalous pathway may at times be blocked. The sinus impulse may then travel anterogradely through the normal pathway only but is able to return retrogradely through the anomalous pathway (Figs. 187B and 190B). It may then travel anterogradely through the normal A-V nodal once again. And if this mechanism continues, a *circus movement* is established between the normal and anomalous A-V pathways resulting in a tachycardia. This is a form of reciprocal rhythm, and the resulting tachycardia is known as a reciprocating tachycardia.

Since anterograde conduction during the tachycardia occurs through the normal A-V nodal pathway only, no delta wave is inscribed. Thus, the typical complex of the W-P-W syndrome disappears during the tachycardia. Furthermore, since the mechanism is a circus movement, it is clear that the tachycardia cannot be complicated by second degree A-V block; any block of the circus movement would immediately terminate the tachycardia.

Note: Supraventricular tachycardias which are not due to the W-P-W syndrome are usually accompanied by second degree A-V block when the rate exceeds 200 beats per minute. The reciprocating tachycardia of the W-P-W syndrome, however, can be conducted without block even when the rate exceeds 200 beats per minute (Fig. 193, lower strip).

B. *Paroxysmal atrial flutter or fibrillation*
The initiation of atrial fibrillation or atrial flutter in the W-P-W syndrome is brought about by the basic reciprocal mechanism facilitated by the by-pass. The by-pass permits the rapid and early return of the supraventricular impulse to the atria; and the returning impulse may,

as a result, reach the atria at the end of their refractory period—during their early simple out-of-phase state or vulnerable phase. Atrial fibrillation or flutter may therefore be precipitated. Since a large atrial mass (as found in acquired heart disease) is necessary to maintain fibrillation or flutter, the fibrillation or flutter of the W-P-W syndrome is rarely maintained for long periods and is consequently paroxysmal in nature.

2. CONDITIONS SIMULATED BY THE W-P-W SYNDROME

The W-P-W syndrome may simulate the following conditions:

A. *Myocardial infarction*

A negative delta wave in Standard lead I and lead AVL may simulate anterolateral myocardial infarction (Fig. 191). A negative delta wave in Standard lead III and lead AVF may simulate inferior myocardial infarction. The tall R waves in the right precordial leads in the Type A W-P-W syndrome may simulate true posterior infarction.

B. *Right ventricular hypertrophy*

The tall R waves in the right precordial leads in the Type A W-P-W syndrome may simulate right ventricular hypertrophy (Fig. 191).

C. *Bundle branch block*

The combination of a prominent delta wave and QRS complex may

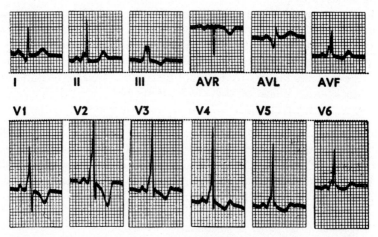

FIG. 191. Electrocardiogram showing the W-P-W syndrome. Note the short P–R interval, delta wave and widened QRS complex—well seen in most leads. The delta wave is negative in Standard lead I and lead AVL and may be mistaken for the pathological Q wave of an anterolateral myocardial infarction.

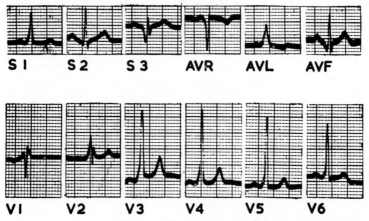

S I   S 2   S 3   AVR   AVL   AVF

V I   V2   V3   V4   V5   V6

FIG. 192. Electrocardiogram showing the W-P-W syndrome. Note the short P–R interval, delta wave and widened QRS complex—well seen in most leads. The delta wave is negative in Standard lead III and AVF and may be mistaken for the pathological Q wave of inferior myocardial infarction.

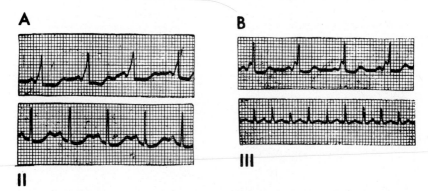

A   B

II   III

FIG. 193. Electrocardiograms A and B are from different patients with the W-P-W syndrome. The upper strips were recorded during slow rates and show the typical QRS pattern, viz. delta wave, widened QRS complex and short P–R interval. The lower strips were recorded from the same patients using the same leads and show the disappearance of the typical QRS pattern during paroxysmal tachycardia.

result in the appearance of a 'notched' QRS complex which may simulate bundle branch block (e.g. leads V1 and V2 in Fig. 192).

D. *Simulated primary myocardial disease*
Secondary S-T segment and T wave changes—S-T segment depression, horizontality, and T wave inversion—may be associated with the abnormal intraventricular depolarization of the W-P-W syndrome. These

secondary S-T segment and T wave changes may be mistaken for the primary S-T segment and T wave changes of myocardial disease (e.g. leads V1 to V6 in Fig. 191).

REFERENCES

1 ROSENBAUM F. F., HECHT H. H., WILSON F. N. & JOHNSTON F. D. (1945) The potential variations of the thorax and the oesophagus in anomalous atrioventricular excitation (Wolff-Parkinson-White syndrome). *Amer. Heart J.* **29**, 281.

2 SODI-PALLARES D. & CALDER R. M. (1956) *New Bases of Electrocardiography.* St. Louis: C. V. Mosby Co.

3 WOLFF L., PARKINSON L. & WHITE P. D. (1930) Bundle branch block with short P–R interval in healthy young people prone to paroxysmal tachycardia. *Amer. Heart J.* **5**, 685.

Dual Rhythms

CHAPTER 20

A-V Dissociation

A-V dissociation is a *non-specific* or *generic* term which may be applied to any rhythm where the atria and the ventricles are activated independently, i.e. by two pacemakers; the atria being governed by one pacemaker, and the ventricles by another. A-V dissociation is not a primary disturbance, and the term, as such, is never a primary diagnosis (Pick, 1953[2]), for the condition always comes about as a result of another arrhythmic disturbance.

BASIC MECHANISMS

There are two basic mechanisms which may lead to A-V dissociation. These are:

1. **A disturbance of impulse formation.**
2. **A disturbance of impulse conduction.**

1. DISTURBANCES OF IMPULSE FORMATION

Disturbances of impulse formation may lead to A-V dissociation if they result in fortuitous, synchronous or near-synchronous discharge of supraventricular and ventricular pacemakers. When this occurs, the impulses from these pacemakers meet or 'collide'—usually within the A-V node, and impede each other's mutual progress. This mutual impedence is termed **interference**, for in an electrical sense, the impulses interfere with each other's conduction. The resulting dissociation is termed **'interference-dissociation'**.

EXAMPLES:

A. *Ventricular or A-V nodal extrasystoles*, where the ventricular or A-V nodal discharge occurs at the same time as the sinus discharge (Figs. 139, 140 and 141).

B. *Ventricular or A-V nodal tachycardia* which are complicated by inter- ference. See section below on interference-dissociation.

C. *A-V nodal or ventricular escape beats* where the escaping focus dis- charges at the same time as the delayed sinus discharge (Figs. 155, 156, 157 and 158).

2. DISTURBANCES OF IMPULSE CONDUCTION

Complete A-V block or high-grade A-V block will lead to A-V disso- ciation since the sinus and subsidiary escape impulses (A-V nodal or ventricular) are prevented from 'invading' each other's territory.

INTERFERENCE-DISSOCIATION

There are two basic disturbances of *impulse formation* which may lead to interference-dissociation. These are:

1. Late or delayed impulse formation.
2. Early or accelerated impulse formation.

1. LATE OR DELAYED IMPULSE FORMATION LEADING TO INTERFERENCE-DISSOCIATION

Interference-dissociation may be brought about by late or delayed impulse formation. For example, the advent of sinus bradycardia may result in a prolongation of the sinus cycle so that it approximates the cycle of a subsidiary A-V nodal or ventricular escape rhythm. When this occurs, the delayed sinus impulse will discharge synchronously with the escaping impulse. The two impulses then meet and interfere with each other's mutual progress, resulting in interference-dissociation (Figs. 155, 156, 157, 158 and 194).

2. PREMATURE OR ENHANCED IMPULSE FORMATION LEADING TO INTERFERENCE-DISSOCIATION

Interference-dissociation may be brought about by premature or enhanced impulse formation of a subsidiary A-V nodal or ventricular pacemaker, e.g. A-V nodal and ventricular extrasystoles (Figs. 136, 139, 140 and 141), idionodal tachycardia (Fig. 138), extrasystolic A-V nodal tachycardia (Fig. 137), idioventricular tachycardia (Figs. 151 and 152), extrasystolic ventricular tachycardia (Figs. 146 and 148). When this occurs, the subsidiary A-V nodal or ventricular cycles may be so shortened that they approximate the sinus cycle. Consequently both the sinus and subsidiary pacemakers discharge synchronously or

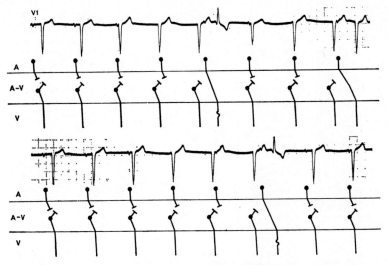

Fig. 194. Electrocardiogram (continuous strip of lead V1) showing *sinus bradycardia* with *A-V dissociation* from an *idionodal escape rhythm*. The P waves of the slower sinus rhythm are dissociated from the QRS complexes of the *relatively* faster idionodal rhythm. The impulses from these two rhythms meet within the A-V node and interfere with, or impede, each other's mutual progress, thereby resulting in A-V dissociation. Since the sinus rhythm is slower than the idionodal rhythm the P waves 'encroach' progressively on the QRS complexes, and then 'overtake'— are recorded after—the QRS complexes. When the sinus impulse occurs after the idionodal beat it may reach the A-V node when it is no longer refractory consequent to activation by the idionodal impulse. When this occurs, the sinus impulse is conducted to, and momentarily activates or captures, the ventricles. There are three capture beats in the recording (diagrammed). The first and third capture beats are conducted with phasic aberrant ventricular conduction resulting in bizarre QRS complexes which are related to the preceding P waves. The second capture beat is conducted with a longer P–R interval thereby resulting in normal intraventricular conduction, since both bundle branches have adequate time for recovery. The QRS complex of the normally conducted capture beat resembles the QRS complexes of the idionodal rhythm thus establishing the A-V nodal origin of the idionodal rhythm.

near-synchronously, and their impulses will meet and interfere with each other's mutual progress within the A-V node.

Note: A-V dissociation will also be facilitated with enhanced subsidiary rhythms if, in addition, there is retrograde A-V block. When this occurs, the faster subsidiary rhythm can co-exist with a much slower sinus rhythm.

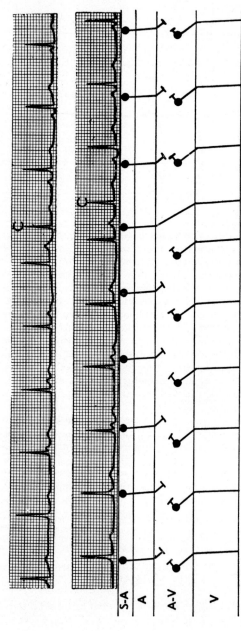

FIG. 195. Electrocardiogram (continuous recording of Standard lead II; the diagram refers to the bottom strip only) showing interference-dissociation. The sinus discharge is slower than the A-V nodal discharge, i.e. the P–P intervals are longer than the R–R intervals; the P waves are thus unrelated to, or dissociated from, the QRS complexes. The first P wave in the lower strip is hidden within the QRS complex; the second P wave deforms the terminal part of the QRS complex; subsequent P waves occur progressively further away from the QRS complexes. The first sinus discharges (lower strip) find the A-V node refractory; the sixth sinus discharge occurs at a relatively longer interval from the preceding QRS complex and thus finds the A-V node recovered; it is therefore conducted to the ventricles resulting in a premature QRS complex—the capture beat (labelled C).

CAPTURE BEATS

When interference-dissociation occurs between sinus rhythm and a faster subsidiary (ventricular or A-V nodal) rhythm, the mutual impedance or interference occurs within the A-V node. The ventricular or A-V nodal impulses cannot be conducted retrogradely to the atria as a result of upper A-V nodal refractoriness consequent to partial penetration of the sinus impulses into the A-V node; and the sinus impulses cannot be conducted anterogradely to the ventricles as a result of lower A-V nodal refractoriness consequent to partial retrograde penetration of the ventricular impulses into the A-V node. However, as the two pacemakers discharge asynchronously, the slower sinus discharge occurs progressively later in relation to the A-V nodal or ventricular discharge, i.e. the sinus P wave 'falls' further and further away from the QRS complex of the subsidiary rhythm. The sinus impulse may thus eventually reach the A-V node when it is no longer refractory. It is then able to penetrate the A-V node and be conducted to and activate the ventricles. This momentary activation of the ventricles by the sinus impulse during A-V dissociation is known as a **ventricular capture beat**—for the sinus impulse momentarily captures the ventricles which are under control of the subsidiary pacemaker. The capture beat occurs before the next scheduled subsidiary beat and is therefore an *early* beat. And this early beat must be related to a preceding sinus P wave (Figs. 148, 194 and 195).

Electrocardiographically the rhythm manifests with P waves which bear no relationship to the QRS complexes. And as the sinus rhythm is slower than the subsidiary ventricular rhythm, the P–P intervals will be longer than the R–R intervals. As a result, the P waves will 'overtake' the QRS complexes, i.e. the 'P–R' interval becomes progressively shorter. The P wave then becomes superimposed upon the QRS complex and eventually occurs after the QRS complex. And when the P wave falls sufficiently far beyond the QRS complex, the sinus impulse is conducted to the ventricles resulting in an earlier QRS complex— the ventricular capture beat.

Note: A-V dissociation should always be suspected when the P–R intervals become progressively shorter.

For further details, the reader is referred to the reviews of Marriott (1958)[1] and Schott (1959).[3]

REFERENCES

1 MARRIOTT H. J. J. (1958) A-V dissociation: a re-appraisal. *Amer. J. Cardiol.* **2,** 586.
2 PICK A. (1963) A-V dissociation. A proposal for a comprehensive classification and consistent terminology. *Amer. Heart J.* **66,** 147.
3 SCHOTT A. (1959) Atrioventricular dissociation with and without interference. *Progr. Cardiovasc. Dis.* **2,** 444.

CHAPTER 21

Parasystole

It is a fundamental law of cardiac physiology that the dominant or fastest pacemaker determines the heart rate. All other subsidiary or slower potential pacemakers are prematurely discharged by the impulses from the dominant pacemaker (see also page 122).

In parasystole, an ectopic pacemaker is in some way *protected* from the impulses of the dominant (usually the sinus) pacemaker. This protective mechanism is situated in the *vicinity of the ectopic focus* and is *operative all the time, viz. throughout the ectopic cycle, i.e. during its refractory phase as well as its non-refractory phase.* The ectopic pacemaker is therefore undisturbed by the sinus impulses and discharges regularly at its own inherent rate. Its discharge will only activate the ventricles and become manifest when it occurs outside the refractory period of the ventricles resulting from their stimulation by the sinus pacemaker. Parasystole is thus a dual rhythm where two pacemakers concurrently and independently govern the heart. The arrhythmia has the following characteristics:

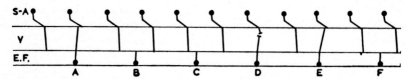

FIG. 196. Diagram illustrating parasystole. The S-A node discharges regularly but its impulse is unable to penetrate the protected ectopic ventricular focus (E.F.). The ectopic focus is thus not disturbed by the sinus rhythm and discharges regularly but at a slower rate than the S-A node. Ectopic impulses B, C and F find the surrounding myocardium refractory after stimulation by the sinus impulse; these discharges are therefore confined to the ectopic focus and are not manifested electrocardiographically. Ectopic impulses A, D and E find the myocardium non-refractory and thus invade the myocardium, becoming manifest. As the ectopic discharge is regular, the longer interectopic interval—A–D—must be a simple multiple of the shortest interectopic interval. D is a fusion complex.

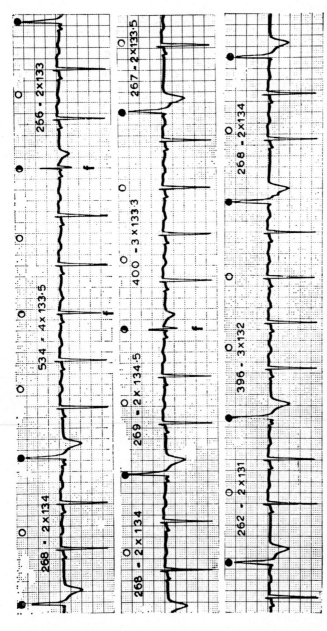

Fig. 197. Electrocardiogram (lead V1) showing ventricular parasystole. *Note*: 1. Marked variation of the coupling intervals between the ectopic (bizarre) beats and the preceding sinus beats. 2. Interectopic intervals which are all in multiples or near-multiples of 1·33 sec. 3. Fusion complexes (labelled f). 4. Black dots indicate manifest ectopic discharges. 5. Open circles indicate non-manifest ectopic discharges. 6. Half-open circles indicate fusion beats.

1. MATHEMATICALLY RELATED INTERECTOPIC INTERVALS

In parasystole some of the ectopic discharges are not manifest since they occur when the ventricles are refractory following activation by the sinus pacemaker. However, the ectopic pacemaker discharges regularly whether its impulses are able to activate the ventricles or not, and thus the longer interectopic intervals—the intervals between manifest ectopic discharges—are multiples of the shortest interectopic interval (Figs. 196 and 197).

2. VARYING COUPLING INTERVALS

The coupling interval is the interval between the ectopic beat and the preceding sinus beat. With ventricular extrasystoles the ectopic beat is in some way forced or precipitated by the preceding sinus beat (Chapter 13); the ectopic beats will thus bear a constant relation to the preceding sinus beats, i.e. the coupling intervals are constant. In parasystole the ectopic pacemaker is autonomous and beats independently of the sinus pacemaker; the two pacemakers beat asynchronously and consequently they have no relationship to each other, i.e. the coupling interval is usually different with each ectopic beat (Fig. 197).

3. FUSION BEATS (ALSO KNOWN AS SUMMATION OR COMBINATION BEATS)

As the two pacemakers in parasystole discharge at their own inherent rates, *occasional*, fortuitous, synchronous or near-synchronous discharge may occur. There will then be simultaneous invasion of the ventricular musculature by both impulses, each activating part of the ventricles. The resulting QRS complex has a configuration intermediate between the 'pure' sinus beat, and the 'pure' ventricular beat. The resulting summation or combination complex is known as a **fusion beat** (Figs. 196 and 197).

SIGNIFICANCE

Parasystole is an uncommon arrhythmia. It may occur with myocardial disease and in association with digitalis administration; but may also occur in normal individuals. The treatment is that of the underlying condition.

PART III

General Considerations

CHAPTER 22

General Considerations

THE APPROACH TO ELECTRO-CARDIOGRAPHIC INTERPRETATION

For adequate electrocardiographic interpretation it is clearly essential to examine every part and aspect of the recording; but perhaps even as important is the necessity to seek out actively the possible abnormal patterns. It is therefore desirable to approach the interpretation of electrocardiograms with specific objectives in mind. The following scheme, while by no means complete, lists some of the important correlative features and abnormal patterns which must be purposefully and specifically looked for in electrocardiographic interpretation.

THE P WAVE

(a) *Atrial enlargement*
   The diagnosis of atrial enlargement is usually best made from the P wave pattern in Standard lead II and lead V1.
(b) *Inverted P waves in Standard leads II and III and lead AVF* suggest retrograde activation of the atria. This may occur, for example, with A-V nodal and ventricular rhythms.
(c) *Inverted P waves in Standard lead I* suggests:
   (i) Incorrect electrode placement (right arm lead attached to left arm, and vice versa).
   (ii) Mirror-image dextrocardia.
   (iii) Possible retrograde atrial activation.

THE P–R INTERVAL

(a) A *prolonged P–R interval* suggests:
   (i) Coronary artery disease   or   (ii) Digitalis effect.
(b) A *short P–R interval* may be due to:
   (i) A dissociated beat.   (iii) A-V nodal rhythm.
   (ii) The W-P-W syndrome.

THE QRS COMPLEX

(a) The diagnosis of *inferior myocardial infarction* is made from the typical infarction pattern—pathological Q wave, raised S-T segment and inverted T wave—in *Standard leads II and III and lead AVF*; leads orientated to the inferior or diaphragmatic surface of the heart.

(*b*) The diagnosis of *anterior myocardial infarction* is made from the typical pattern—pathological Q wave, raised S-T segment and inverted T wave in the *V leads, Standard lead I and lead AVL.*

(*c*) The diagnosis of *right bundle branch block* is usually made from the presence of an rSR' or 'M'-shaped QRS complex in leads V1 and V2.

(*d*) The diagnosis of *left bundle branch* is usually made from the presence of a notched and widened 'M'-shaped QRS complex in leads V5 and V6.

(*e*) *Right ventricular hypertrophy* is usually suggested to tall R waves in leads V1 and V2 and right axis deviation.

(*f*) *Left ventricular hypertrophy* is usually suggested by tall R waves in leads V5 and V6 associated with deep S waves in leads V1 and V2. This may be associated with a 'strain' pattern: depressed convex-upward S-T segments in leads V5 and V6.

THE S-T SEGMENT

(*a*) *Coronary artery disease* is suggested by horizontality, plane depression or sagging of the S-T segment particularly in Standard lead II and leads V5 and V6.

(*b*) *Digitalis effect* is suggested by a mirror-image correction mark shape of the S-T segment—usually seen in leads V5 and V6.

(*c*) *The 'strain pattern'*—depressed convex-upward S-T segment with inverted T wave—may be seen in leads V5 and V6 in left ventricular hypertrophy; and in leads V1 and V2 in right ventricular hypertrophy.

(*d*) *The hyperacute phase* of myocardial infarction and the variant form of angina pectoris (Prinzmetal's Angina) is reflected by slope-elevation of the S-T segment associated with a tall and widened T wave.

THE T WAVE

(*a*) Low or inverted T waves in most leads may be associated with coronary artery disease.

(*b*) Low or inverted T waves associated with generalized low voltage of the QRS complex suggest pericardial effusion or myxoedema.

(*c*) Tall peaked T waves in the precordial leads may be due to:
    (i) Acute subendocardial ischaemia or infarction.
    (ii) Recovering inferior infarction.
    (iii) Hyperkalaemia.

THE U WAVE

(a) An *inverted U wave* in Standard leads I and II, and leads V5 and V6 is usually due to:
   (i) Coronary artery disease,
or
   (ii) Hypertensive heart disease.
(b) A *prominent U wave* in the mid-precordial leads—(V3–V5)—is commonly due to hypopotassaemia.

THE Q–T INTERVAL

The Q–T interval is measured from the *beginning* of the QRS complex (irrespective of whether it begins with a q or r wave) to the *end* of the T wave. It represents the combined phases of depolarization and repolarization.

   The Q–T interval varies with age, sex and rate. It lengthens with bradycardia and shortens with tachycardia; the valid Q–T interval is therefore derived by correcting for the variation in rate. The corrected Q–T interval is known as the QTc, for which absolute values have been established. It must be emphasized, however, that measurement of the Q–T interval is technically difficult and often erroneous. This is due to difficulty in determining the exact end-point of the T wave, since the T wave is often obscured by the U wave. The U wave is, however, usually isoelectric in lead AVL, and it is therefore best to measure the Q–T interval in this lead. The criteria now used for normal and abnormal Q–T intervals are thus only approximate. As a rough guide, the Q–T interval does not normally exceed 0.38 sec at normal heart rates, between 60 and 80 beats per minute, i.e. it should not exceed half the R–R interval.

A prolonged Q–T interval may be associated with:
   Diffuse myocardial disease
   Myocardial infarction
   Acute carditis (e.g. acute rheumatic fever)
   Head injury or cerebrovascular accident
   Hypocalcaemia
   Quinidine effect
   Procaine amide effect
   Cardiac syncope.

A shortened Q–T interval may be associated with:
   Digitalis effect
   Hypercalcaemia.

COMMON ASSOCIATIONS

Electrocardiographic Combinations	*Suggested Diagnosis*

1. Atrial fibrillation
   Right axis deviation
   } Mitral stenosis

2. 'Left atrial' P wave
   Right axis deviation
   } Mitral stenosis

3. Atrial fibrillation
   Right axis deviation
   Left ventricular diastolic
   overload
   } Mitral incompetence

4. *Very tall* 'right atrial' P waves
   First degree A-V block
   Normal QRS axis
   } Tricuspid stenosis

5. 'Left atrial' P wave
   Left ventricular systolic overload
   } Hypertensive heart disease

SOME COMMON ELECTROCARDIOGRAPHIC MANIFESTATIONS OF CONGENITAL HEART DISEASE

Pulmonary Stenosis. The Tetralogy of Fallot

1. *P. congenitale.*
2. Right ventricular systolic overload: *very tall* R waves and S-T segment 'strain' pattern (depressed convex-upward S-T segments and inverted T waves) in leads orientated to the right ventricle—leads V1 to V3 (Fig. 73).
3. Right axis deviation.

Tricuspid Atresia

1. Left axis deviation.
2. Left ventricular dominance.

Note: Most cases of cyanotic congenital heart disease manifest with right ventricular dominance and right axis deviation; tricuspid atresia is a notable exception.

Atrial Septal Defect

Ostium secundum type

1. *Incomplete* or complete right bundle branch block.
2. 1st degree A-V block.

Ostium primum type and *persistent A-V communis*

1. Incomplete or complete right bundle branch block.
2. *Left axis deviation* of the initial vector.

Ventricular Septal Defect (Fig. 198)

1. *Biventricular hypertrophy*:

Right ventricular hypertrophy—right ventricular systolic overload.

Left ventricular hypertrophy—deep S waves over right precordial leads; tall R waves over left precordial leads.

This results in large amplitude diphasic QRS complexes in many leads and is known as the *Katz-Wachtel Phenomenon*.

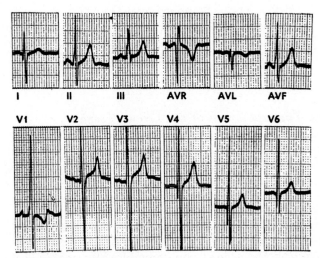

FIG. 198. Electrocardiogram illustrating the features commonly associated with ventricular septal defect. Note (*a*) evidence of right ventricular hypertrophy—tall R waves in leads V1 to V3; (*b*) evidence of left ventricular diastolic overload—tall R waves in leads V4 to V6, deep S waves in leads V2 and V3, *deep Q waves* in leads V4 to V6, and rather tall symmetrical T waves in leads V4 to V6; (*c*) the resultant large amplitude diphasic QRS complexes in Standard leads I, II, leads AVR, AVF and leads V2 to V5—the *Katz-Wachtel Phenomenon*. Note the small initial slur in lead V1.

2. Deep Q waves (associated with tall R waves) over the left precordial leads—leads V5 and V6—are particularly suggestive of ventricular septal defect.

Patent Ductus Arteriosus

This condition is usually manifested by left ventricular diastolic overload.

Ventricular Septal Defect ⎫ **complicated by**
Atrial Septal Defect ⎬ **PULMONARY**
Patent Ductus Arteriosus ⎭ **HYPERTENSION**

The characteristic electrocardiographic features disappear and the main electrocardiographic manifestation is that of right ventricular dominance.

Coarctation of the Aorta
Left ventricular systolic overload.

Ebstein's Anomaly
1. Tall peaked P waves in Standard lead II.
2. Right bundle branch block with small amplitude QRS complexes.
3. Wolff-Parkinson-White syndrome—Type B, i.e. the QRS complex is negative over the right precordial leads (Sodi-Pallares & Calder, 1956[1]).
4. Paroxysmal supraventricular tachycardia.

Corrected Transposition of the Great Vessels
This condition is frequently associated with *A-V dissociation* due to high-grade A-V block. Thus, the combination of A-V dissociation and a pansystolic murmur in a young child is presumptive evidence of possible corrected transposition of the great vessels.

'Mirror-Image' Destrocardia
1. Inverted P waves in Standard lead I (see also page 115).
2. All other deflections—QRS complex and T wave—are negative in Standard lead I; this lead now resembles a normal lead AVR.
3. The normal appearances of Standard leads II and III are interchanged.

Anomalous Left Coronary Artery
When the left coronary artery arises from the pulmonary artery the electrocardiogram reflects the patterns of *anterolateral infarction*, viz. pathological Q waves, raised and coved S-T segments, and inverted T waves in Standard lead I, lead AVL and the left precordial leads.

AN APPROACH TO THE DIAGNOSIS
ARRHYTHMIAS

One of the more important aspects to the solution of an arrhythmia is the *behaviour of the P wave*. This is best seen in Standard lead II or lead VI; at times, special leads have to be used, viz. lead S5* or an oesophageal

---

* The selector switch is set at S1; the right arm—negative—electrode is placed over the manubrium, and the left arm—positive—electrode is placed over the right fifth interspace adjacent to the sternum.

lead. The following procedure is recommended in the study of an arrhythmia.

1. Note the rate of the sinus discharge, i.e. the frequency of the P–P intervals. A rate exceeding 150 per minute in the adult usually, but not invariably, indicates a paroxysmal atrial tachycardia.
2. Note the rhythm or regularity of the P waves:
    (a) A *gradual* increase and diminution of the P–P intervals is characteristic of sinus arrhythmia.
    (b) A *sudden early P wave of different contour* denotes an atrial extrasystole. Note whether this is followed by a normal or aberrant QRS complex, or whether it is not followed by a QRS complex at all—a blocked atrial extrasystole.
3. If typical P waves cannot be identified, note whether the baseline has the 'saw-tooth' appearance of atrial flutter or the chaotic appearance of atrial fibrillation.
4. Note whether each P wave is followed by a QRS complex. If a P wave is not followed by a QRS complex, it may be due to (a) 2nd degree A-V block, in which case all the P–P intervals will be regular (allowing for possible sinus arrhythmia) or (b) a blocked atrial extrasystole, in which case the P wave related to the pause is premature and bizarre. Note that a blocked atrial extrasystole may be superimposed on the preceding T wave and consequently obscured; the situation may then mimic, and be mistaken for, S-A block. The T waves of all pauses must therefore be carefully scrutinized for deformity—no matter how slight.
   Note the duration of the P–R interval. In the case of 2nd degree A-V block, note whether the dropped beat is preceded by a gradual lengthening of the P–R intervals—the Wenckebach Phenomenon.
5. Note whether the beat following a pause is a normal sinus beat or an atrial, A-V nodal, or ventricular, escape beat.
6. If the P waves are not related to the QRS complexes, A-V dissociation is present. This may be due to:
    (a) *Paroxysmal ventricular tachycardia*: the QRS complexes will be bizarre and slightly irregular.
    (b) *Non-paroxysmal or paroxysmal, nodal tachycardia*: the QRS complexes are usually normal in shape.
    Dissociation may be incomplete in any of the above conditions: the rhythm is complicated by capture beats, i.e. interference-dissociation. This is characterized by a *sudden early beat* which is *related to a P wave*.
    (c) *Complete A-V block*: The QRS complexes may be normal or aberrant and are usually recorded at a rate of less than 40 per minute.
7. An arrhythmia with a bizarre QRS pattern does not necessarily

connote an ectopic ventricular origin, but may be due to *Phasic Aberrant Ventricular Conduction*; in such instances, the relationship of the P wave to the QRS complex and the contour of the QRS complex (particularly in lead V1 and the other precordial leads) will usually indicate the correct diagnosis.

Examples:

(a) An early bizarre QRS complex during normal sinus rhythm may, at first glance, be mistaken for a ventricular extrasystole. If, however, it is preceded by a premature and abnormal P wave, it is due to an atrial extrasystole with phasic aberrant ventricular conduction.

(b) A rapid rhythm characterized by repeated bizarre QRS complexes may be due to:

(i) Supraventricular tachycardia with phasic aberrant ventricular conduction: *all* the bizarre QRS complexes will be preceded by P waves.

(ii) Paroxysmal ventricular tachycardia. The bizarre QRS complexes may be completely dissociated from the P waves (the rhythm may also be complicated by possible capture beats). When the ectopic ventricular impulses are conducted retrogradely to the atria, each QRS complex will be related to an ensuing P wave. When the QRS:P relationship cannot be established with certainty, the contour of the QRS complex in the precordial leads, particularly lead V1 (or MCL1), may indicate the correct diagnosis (see Chapter 18, page 188).

SOME FURTHER OBSERVATIONS ON ABNORMAL RHYTHMS

A SLOW REGULAR VENTRICULAR RHYTHM may be due to:

1. Sinus bradycardia
2. Complete A-V block with idioventricular rhythm
3. 2:1 A-V block
4. 2:1 S-A block (very rare)
5. Atrial flutter with high-grade (e.g. 4:1) A-V block
6. Idionodal escape rhythm
7. Idioventricular escape rhythm.

Causes of
IRREGULAR VENTRICULAR RHYTHM

1. Atrial fibrillation
2. Irregularly occurring atrial and/or ventricular extrasystoles

3. Atrial flutter with varying 2nd degree A-V block
4. Paroxysmal atrial tachycardia with varying 2nd degree A-V block
5. *Marked* respiratory sinus arrhythmia.

'SLOW' ATRIAL FIBRILLATION

'Slow' atrial fibrillation usually reflects treatment with digitalis. A more correct description is—atrial fibrillation with slow or diminished ventricular response.

SOME COMMON CAUSES OF BIGEMINAL RHYTHM

Alternate ventricular extrasystoles (common)
Alternate atrial or nodal extrasystoles
3:2 A-V block
Atrial flutter with alternating 4:1 and 2:1 A-V block.

ABSENT P WAVES

Absent P waves may be due to:
1. S-A block
2. Atrial fibrillation
3. Hyperkalaemia
4. A-V nodal rhythm (the P waves may be hidden within the QRS complexes).

A LONG PAUSE interrupting regular rhythm may be caused by:
1. A 'dropped beat' as a result of second degree A-V block
2. A 'dropped beat' as a result of S-A block
3. A blocked or non-conducted atrial extrasystole.

When the P–R INTERVAL BECOMES PROGRESSIVELY SHORTER, A-V DISSOCIATION is usually present.

EXTRASYSTOLES occur PREMATURELY; ESCAPE BEATS occur LATE.

PAROXYSMAL ATRIAL RHYTHM (tachycardia, paroxysmal or flutter fibrillation) in a young person without obvious evidence of cardiac disease raises the possibility of:
1. Thyrotoxicosis
2. The W-P-W syndrome.

SOME OTHER ASPECTS

TALL SYMMETRICAL T WAVES IN THE PRECORDIAL LEADS

These may be due to:
1. Acute subendocardial ischaemia, injury or infarction
2. Recovering inferior infarction
3. Hyperkalaemia.

GENERALIZED LOW VOLTAGE

This may be due to:
1. Incorrect standardization
2. Emphysema
3. Obesity or thick chest wall
4. Pericardial effusion or constrictive pericarditis
5. Myxoedema.

ACUTE RHEUMATIC FEVER

This is frequently associated with:
1. Sinus tachycardia
2. Non-paroxysmal A-V nodal tachycardia—idionodal tachycardia
3. Prolonged P–R interval
4. Second degree A-V block
5. Prolonged Q–T interval.

THE TRANSITION ZONE

The precordial transition zone characterizes the transition from the rS complexes, recorded by leads orientated to the right ventricle, to the qR complexes, recorded by leads orientated to the left ventricle. This zone is usually reflected by lead V3 or lead V4. The complexes in these leads are usually intermediate in shape between the typical rS and qR configurations, and the T waves may be notched or bifid. This zone is therefore characterized by atypical or even bizarre deflections and caution should be exercised in interpreting abnormality solely from these leads.

Electrocardiographic abnormalities may occur in normal healthy persons and in the absence of organic heart disease.

Organic heart disease may occur with normal electrocardiographic patterns.

Serial electrocardiographic studies are of particular value, as a changing pattern is usually significant.

Inquiry should always be made whether the patient has been taking drugs. Digitalis is the arch-simulator and may mimic almost any abnormal electrocardiographic pattern.

The electrocardiogram is only a supplementary aid to diagnosis and must always be used by the clinician in conjunction with the clinical examination.

REFERENCE

1 SODI-PALLARES D. & CALDER R. M. (1956) *New Bases of Electrocardiography.* St. Louis: C. V. Mosby and Co.

FORM FOR ROUTINE REPORTING

Name: ....   Date: ....
Age: ....   Registration No.: ....
Drugs: ....   Ward and Bed No.: ....

Rate:	e.g. 140 per minute
Rhythm:	e.g. sinus arrhythmia
P wave:	e.g. tall and peaked in Standard lead II and lead V1
P–R interval:	e.g. 0.26 second
QRS complex:	
Width	e.g. 0.12 second in lead V1
Axis	e.g. −30°
Configuration.........	e.g. normal
	or
	deep Q waves in leads ....
	or
	R–R complex in leads ....
	or
	tall R waves in leads ....
	or
	deep S waves in leads ....
S-T segment:	e.g. coved
	raised } in leads ....
	plane depression
T wave:	low to inverted throughout
	or
	tall and symmetrical in leads ....
U wave:	e.g. inverted in leads ....
	or
	prominent in leads ....
Comments:	List abnormalities here
1.	e.g. 1. *P. mitrale*
2.	2. first degree A-V block
3.	3. right axis deviation
4.	4. right ventricular systolic overload
	or
5.	e.g. 1. atrial fibrillation
6.	2. right bundle branch block
Conclusions:	*Suggested terminology:*
	1. Normal electrocardiogram.
	2. The electrocardiogram is within normal limits.

3. Borderline electrocardiogram (list questionable features).
4. Abnormal electrocardiogram characteristic (or diagnostic) of ....
5. Abnormal electrocardiogram suggestive of ....
6. Abnormal electrocardiogram consistent with ....
7. Abnormal non-specific electrocardiogram (list abnormal features).

Additional remarks:

1. Suggest serial records
2. Suggest additional leads
3. Record Standard lead III in deep inspiration and deep expiration
4. Suggest exercise test

Electrocardiographic Measurements

(Fig. 199)

1. The **P–R interval** is measured from the *beginning* of the P wave to the *beginning* of the QRS complex irrespective of whether the QRS complex begins with a Q or an R wave.
2. The **Q–T interval** is measured from the *beginning* of the QRS complex to the *end* of the T wave.
3. The **intrinsicoid deflection** begins after the maximum QRS deflection has been inscribed, i.e. at the *peak of the R wave in qR complexes*, and at the *lowest point of the S wave in rS complexes*.
4. The **ventricular activation time—VAT**—is the interval between the beginning of the QRS complex and the onset of the intrinsicoid deflection.

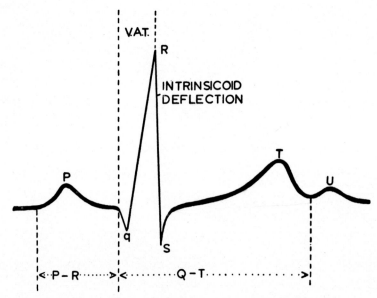

FIG. 199. Diagram illustrating various electrocardiographic measurements.

ELEMENTARY ELECTROPHYSIOLOGY

In a healthy resting muscle cell, certain molecules dissociate into positive and negative ions. The positively charged ions are on the outer surface, and the negatively charged ions on the inner surface, of the cell membrane (Figs. 200 and 202). The positive charges are exactly equal in number to the negative charges; the cell is in a state of electrical balance and is said to be **polarized**.

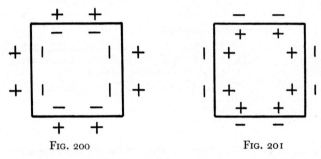

Fig. 200. Diagram illustrating a polarized or resting cell.

Fig. 201. Diagram illustrating a depolarized or activated cell.

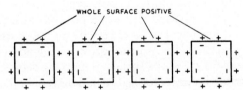

Fig. 202. Diagram illustrating polarized or resting cardiac muscle. All cells have positive surface charges.

Note: When two electrical charges of equal and opposite direction, i.e. one positive ion and one negative ion, are juxtaposed on either side of a membrane, they constitute a **Dipole** (Fig. 203).

When two charged ions of equal and opposite direction are situated *next to each other on the surface of an excitable tissue,* they constitute a **Doublet** (Fig. 203). The term 'doublet' was introduced by Craib (1927)[1] to distinguish it from the dipole.

When the cell is *stimulated* or *injured,* the negative ions migrate to the outer surface of the cell and the positive charges pass into the cell, i.e. the polarity is reversed. This process is termed depolarization (Figs. 201 and 203). With recovery, positive charges return to the outer surface and negative charges migrate into the cell. This process is termed repolarization, i.e. the polarity or electrical balance of the cell is re-established.

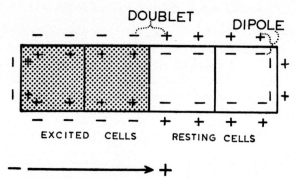

FIG. 203. Diagram illustrating the passage of excitation through a potentially excitable tissue. Note (a) excited cells—shaded area; the surface is electrically negative; (b) resting cells—the surface is electrically positive; (c) a *Dipole*—a pair of opposite charges on either side of the cell membrane; (d) a *Doublet*—a pair of adjacent but opposite charges on the surface of the membrane.

A series of cells in the resting state will all have positive surface charges; no difference in electrical potential exists and no current flows (Fig. 202).

If a stimulus travels through these resting (polarized) cells, those cells initially activated or depolarized will have negative surface charges whilst those not yet activated will have positive surface charges (Fig. 203). A potential electrical difference will therefore exist between the *surface* of the excitable cells and the *surface* of the adjacent resting cells and a current will flow, i.e. the surface boundary between excitable and non-excitable tissue is characterized by a doublet. And as a doublet will always exist between the surfaces of excited and resting cells, *the flow of an electrical current may be viewed as a series of doublets* (Craib, 1927[1]).

This current will have a positive 'head' and a negative 'tail'. A unipolar electrode, or positive pole of a bipolar electrode, orientated towards the oncoming 'head' will record a positive or upward deflection; a unipolar electrode, or negative pole of a bipolar electrode, orientated towards the receding 'tail' will record a negative or downward deflection (Fig. 1).

THE CURRENT OF INJURY

Injured myocardial tissue is reflected by a raised S-T segment in leads orientated to the injured surface, and by a depressed S-T segment in leads orientated to the uninjured surface. The mechanism governing this manifestation has not, as yet, been fully elucidated. One of the postulates is presented below.

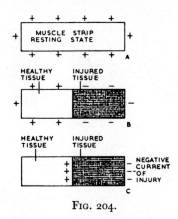

FIG. 204.

Mechanism

Resting healthy myocardium has an electrically positive surface charge. When the whole muscle is in a resting state, all the surface charges are positive, no difference of electrical potential exists on the surface, and there is therefore no flow of current (Fig. 204A).

When heart muscle is either *stimulated* or *injured* its surface becomes electrically negative (see page 227, Fig. 203). If only part of a muscle strip is injured (Figs. 204B and 210), the injured part will have a negative surface charge and the adjacent healthy muscle will have a positive surface charge. This surface difference in potential between the injured and uninjured tissues leads to a flow of current. (See also Craib's 'doublet concept'— page 228.) Thus, in effect, when a portion of heart muscle is injured, a continuous negative current—the current of injury —is emitted from the injured surface while a continuous positive current is emitted from the side of the injured tissue adjacent to the healthy muscle (Figs 204C and 210A).

When the ventricle is injured as a result of myocardial infarction, a layer of muscle immediately adjacent to the endocardial surface is usually spared (Figs. 205 to 209; see also Fig. 23).

Thus an infarct of the left ventricular wall which causes injury but not death of tissue will emit a continuous negative current to an electrode orientated to the left ventricle, and this is recorded as a depressed

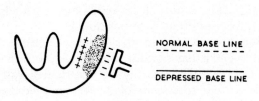

FIG. 205.

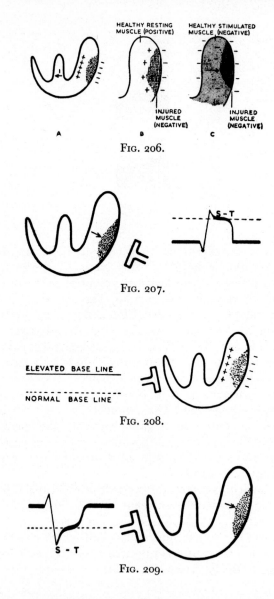

FIG. 206.

FIG. 207.

FIG. 208.

FIG. 209.

baseline (Fig. 205). This is also illustrated in Fig. 210A where the baseline is depressed from position X to position Y.

Depolarization now occurs in the usual way from left to right through the interventricular septum (Fig. 206A), and then from right to left through the remaining healthy left ventricular wall (Fig. 206C).

As previously stated, *stimulation* of healthy muscle tissue will also result in a negative surface charge. Thus, after depolarization of the healthy part of the left ventricular wall, the healthy but stimulated tissue will also have a negative surface charge (Figs. 206C and 210B).

Since all surface charges have become electrically negative (i.e. of both the healthy stimulated tissue and the injured tissue), a potential difference no longer exists, no current flows and the continuous negative current of injury is abolished. As a result, the depressed baseline returns to the normal level giving the impression of a raised S-T segment (Figs. 207 and 210B). When the healthy stimulated muscle returns to the resting state, the negative current of injury reappears and the baseline is again depressed (Fig. 210C).

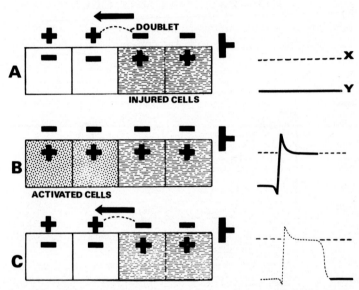

FIG. 210. Diagrams illustrating the effects of myocardial injury: the current injury.

The myocardial injury is reflected by a **raised S-T segment in leads orientated to the injured surface**. The S-T is also **coved**, i.e. convex upwards (e.g. lead V2–V6 in Fig. 28).

Conversely, an electrode facing the uninjured surface will record an elevated baseline due to the continuous emission of a positive current (Fig. 208).

During depolarization of the remaining healthy part of the left ventricle, the continuous positive force (directed to leads facing the uninjured surface) is abolished in a manner analogous to that described above. Consequently the baseline momentarily returns to normal, giving the impression of a depressed S-T segment (e.g. lead AVL in Fig. 36).

THE TRANSMEMBRANE ACTION POTENTIAL

The electrocardiogram reflects the electrical activity of cardiac tissue. The electrical activity of a single muscle cell can be reflected experimentally by an intracellular micro-electrode which records the potential differences between it and an external reference electrode. The record is termed the **monophasic action potential** or the **transmembrane action potential**.

THE ACTION POTENTIAL OF A
NON-PACEMAKING CELL

The resting potential of a myocardial cell is negative with respect to an external reference electrode and, by convention, is labelled phase 4

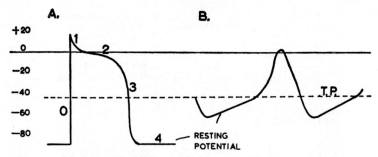

FIG. 211. Diagrams illustrating A. Action potential of a non-pacemaking cell, and B. Action potential of a pacemaking cell.

(Diagram A of Fig. 211). The resting potential of a non-pacemaking cell is stable, i.e. it remains at a constant, 'horizontal', negative, sub-threshold level until depolarization by a propagated impulse results in its abrupt reversal, i.e. it becomes positive. The activated or excited state is termed the action potential (Diagram A of Fig. 211).

In common with all other types of excitable cells, the action potential of a non-pacemaking cardiac cell begins with an initial rapid depolarization—an abrupt upstroke which is labelled *Phase* o (Diagram A of Fig. 211). The action potential of cardiac cells differs from that of other excitable cells in exhibiting a slow delayed repolarization which may be divided into three phases:

Phase 1: a phase of early and rapid repolarization.
Phase 2: a phase of slow repolarization—termed *the plateau*.
Phase 3: a terminal phase of relatively rapid repolarization.

During the terminal phase of depolarization (Phase o), as well as during the early stages of repolarization (Phase 1 and the early part of Phase 2), the inside of the cell becomes temporarily positive in relation to the outside. This is termed the *overshoot* or *reversal*, and is represented in Diagram A of Fig. 211 by that part of the action potential which is situated above the zero level.

THE ACTION POTENTIAL OF A PACEMAKING CELL

The action potential of a pacemaking cell differs from that of a non-pacemaking cell in several respects (Diagram B of Fig. 211). The velocity of the upstroke of Phase 0 is somewhat slower. The reversal is small or absent. The peak is rounded. Phase 2 has a steeper decline and therefore does not usually exhibit the characteristic plateau configuration. The magnitude—or 'depth'—of the resting potential is less than that found with non-pacemaking cells. The most characteristic feature of a pacemaking cell, however, and its most striking difference from a non-pacemaking cell, is the presence of **slow spontaneous depolarization during Phase 4—diastolic depolarization.** The record reveals a 'resting' potential that exhibits a gradual upward slope. This slow diastolic depolarization begins immediately after Phase 3 resulting in a gradual loss of resting potential, i.e. the resting potential becomes less negative; and when the resting potential is reduced to a critical threshold level, there is a *smooth* but rapid transition to the upstroke of Phase 0 (Draper & Weidemann, 1951[2]).

The effect of diastolic depolarization is that the resting potential *regularly* and *automatically* reaches threshold level, thereby resulting in a regular, spontaneous, automatic discharge. Thus, diastolic depolariza-

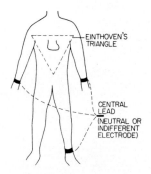

FIG. 212. Diagram illustrating the deviation of the neutral limb of a unipolar electrode. Note the three limb electrodes are joined to form a single lead—the neutral or indifferent lead.

tion reflects a pacemaking property—the property of automaticity or rhythmicity.

THE DERIVATION OF UNIPOLAR LEADS

The heart may be considered to lie in the centre of an equilateral triangle formed by the Standard leads (see Chapter 7 and Figs. 95 and 96). The apices of this triangle are thus, in a sense, the right arm, left arm and left leg electrodes (Fig. 212; see also Figs. 95 and 96). According to Einthoven, the sum of the potentials of these three leads is at any instant equal to zero. Thus, if these three leads are connected to a central terminal, the potential of this terminal will be zero (Fig. 212).

If this central terminal (also termed the neutral or indifferent electrode) is connected to one pole of the galvanometer, that lead will always have a potential value of zero. The electrode connected to the other pole of the galvanometer will record the true potential at any given point. This electrode is termed the exploring electrode (Fig. 213).

The development of this lead is due mainly to the work of Wilson and his associates (1944).[4]

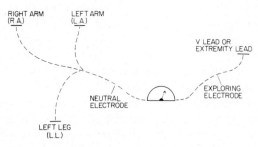

FIG. 213. Diagram illustrating the deviation of a unipolar lead. The neutral limb is connected to the negative pole of the galvanometer; the exploring electrode is connected to the positive pole of the galvanometer.

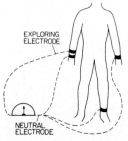

FIG. 214. Diagram illustrating the derivation of lead VR. Note that the right arm has connections from both the neutral and exploring electrodes.

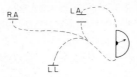

FIG. 215. Diagram illustrating the derivation of lead VL. Note that the left arm has connections from both the neutral and exploring electrodes.

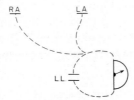

FIG. 216. Diagram illustrating the derivation of lead VF. Note that the left leg has connections from both the neutral and exploring electrodes.

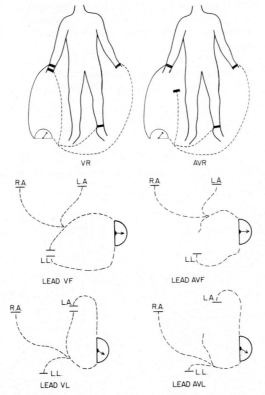

FIG. 217. Diagrams illustrating the derivation of leads AVR, AVL, and AVF.

EXTREMITY LEADS

Lead VR is obtained by connecting the exploring electrode to the right arm (Fig. 214).

Lead VL is obtained by connecting the exploring electrode to the left arm (Fig. 215).

Lead VF is obtained by connecting the exploring electrode to the left leg (Fig. 216).

Using the above technique, the potential obtained by the exploring electrode is of low voltage. Goldberger (1942)[3] augmented this voltage by omitting the connection of the neutral terminal to the limb which is being tested and allowing it to hang free (Fig. 217). The addition of the letter A is used to designate the augmented lead.

REFERENCES

1   CRAIB W. H. (1927) A study of the electrical field surrounding heart muscle. *Heart* **14,** 71.

2   DRAPER M. H. & WEIDEMANN S. (1951) Cardiac resting action potentials recorded with an intracellular electrode. *J. Physiol. (Lond.)* **155,** 74.

3   GOLDBERGER E. (1942) A simple indifferent, electrocardiographic electrode of zero potential and a technique of obtaining augmented, unipolar, extremity leads. *Amer. Heart J.* **23,** 483.

4   WILSON F. N., JOHNSTON F. D., ROSENBAUM F., ERLANDER H., KOSSMAN C., HECHT H., COTRIM N., MENEZES DE OLIVEIRA R., SCARSI R. & BARKER P. S. (1944) The precordial electrocardiogram. *Amer. Heart J.* **27,** 19.

Index